W9-CZK-607

Regional Analgesia and Acute Pain Management

Guest Editors

SUGANTHA GANAPATHY, MBBS
VINCENT CHAN, MD

ANESTHESIOLOGY CLINICS

www.anesthesiology.theclinics.com

Consulting Editor
LEE A. FLEISHER, MD, FACC

June 2011 • Volume 29 • Number 2

SAUNDERS an imprint of ELSEVIER, Inc.

W.B. SAUNDERS COMPANY

A Division of Elsevier Inc.

1600 John F. Kennedy Boulevard, Suite 1800 • Philadelphia, PA 19103-2899

http://www.theclinics.com

ANESTHESIOLOGY CLINICS Volume 29, Number 2
June 2011 ISSN 1932-2275, ISBN-13: 978-1-4377-2426-4

Editor: Rachel Glover
Developmental Editor: Donald Mumford

Anesthesiology Clinics (ISSN 1932-2275) is published quarterly by Elsevier Inc., 360 Park Avenue South, New York, NY 10010-1710. Months of issue are March, June, September, and December. Periodicals postage paid at New York, NY and at additional mailing offices. Subscription prices are $141.00 per year (US student/resident), $287.00 per year (US individuals), $351.00 per year (Canadian individuals), $459.00 per year (US institutions), $569.00 per year (Canadian institutions), $198.00 per year (Canadian and foreign student/resident), $398.00 per year (foreign individuals), and $569.00 per year (foreign institutions). To receive student and resident rate, orders must be accompanied by name of affiliated institution, date of term, and the *signature* of program/residency coordinator on institutions letterhead. Orders will be billed at individual rate until proof of status is received. Foreign air speed delivery is included in all *Clinics'* subscription prices. All prices are subject to change without notice. POSTMASTER: Send address changes to *Anesthesiology Clinics,* Elsevier Health Sciences Division, Subscription Customer Service, 3251 Riverport Lane, Maryland Heights, MO 63043. Customer Service (orders, claims, online, change of address): Elsevier Health Sciences Division, Subscription Customer Service, 3251 Riverport Lane, Maryland Heights, MO 63043. Tel:1-800-654-2452 (U.S. and Canada); 314-447-8871 (outside U.S. and Canada). Fax: 314-447-8029. E-mail: journalscustomerservice-usa@elsevier.com (for print support); journalsonlinesupport-usa@elsevier.com (for online support).

Reprints. For copies of 100 or more of articles in this publication, please contact the Commercial Reprints Department, Elsevier Inc., 360 Park Avenue South, New York, NY 10010-1710. Tel.: 212-633-3812; Fax: 212-462-1935; E-mail: reprints@elsevier.com.

Anesthesiology Clinics, is also published in Spanish by McGraw-Hill Inter-americana Editores S. A., P.O. Box 5-237, 06500 Mexico D. F., Mexico.

Anesthesiology Clinics, is covered in *MEDLINE/PubMed (Index Medicus), Current Contents/Clinical Medicine, Excerpta Medica, ISI/BIOMED,* and *Chemical Abstracts.*

Printed in the United States of America.

Contributors

CONSULTING EDITOR

LEE A. FLEISHER, MD, FACC
Robert D. Dripps Professor and Chair of Anesthesiology and Critical Care, University of Pennsylvania School of Medicine, Philadelphia, Pennsylvania

GUEST EDITORS

SUGANTHA GANAPATHY, MBBS, DA, FRCA, FFARCS (I), FRCPC
Professor of Anesthesiology and Perioperative Medicine, Director of Regional and Pain Research, Department of Anesthesiology and Perioperative Medicine, London Health Sciences Centre, University Hospital, University of Western Ontario, London, Ontario, Canada; Consulting Professor, Duke University Medical Centre, Durham, North Carolina

VINCENT CHAN, MD, FRCPC
Professor, Department of Anesthesiology, University of Toronto, Toronto Western Hospital, Toronto, Ontario, Canada

AUTHORS

JOSÉ AGUIRRE, MD
Consultant, Department of Anesthesiology, Balgrist University Hospital, Zurich, Switzerland

JOHN G. ANTONAKAKIS, MD
Staff Anesthesiologist, Portsmouth Anesthesia Associates, Portsmouth Regional Hospital, Portsmouth, New Hampshire

ALAIN BORGEAT, MD
Professor and Chief-of-Staff, Department of Anesthesiology, Balgrist University Hospital, Zurich, Switzerland

ROBERT BOURNE, MD, FRCSC
Professor, Division of Orthopedics, Department of Surgery, University of Western Ontario, London, Ontario, Canada

JONATHAN BROOKES, FRCA
Clinical Fellow in Regional Anesthesia, University of Western Ontario, London, Ontario, Canada

MARC DE KOCK, MD, PhD
Department of Anesthesia and Perioperative Medicine, Catholic University of Louvain, St Luc Hospital, Brussels, Belgium

SUGANTHA GANAPATHY, MBBS, DA, FRCA, FFARCS (I), FRCPC
Professor of Anesthesiology and Perioperative Medicine, Director of Regional and Pain Research, Department of Anesthesiology and Perioperative Medicine, London Health Sciences Centre, University Hospital, University of Western Ontario, London, Ontario, Canada; Consulting Professor, Duke University Medical Centre, Durham, North Carolina

KISHOR GANDHI, MD, MPH
Director, Regional Anesthesia and Assistant Professor of Anesthesiology, Thomas Jefferson University, Jefferson Medical College, Philadelphia, Pennsylvania

IRINA GROSU, MD
Department of Anesthesia and Perioperative Medicine, Catholic University of Louvain, St Luc Hospital, Brussels, Belgium

JAMES W. HEITZ, MD, FACP
Director, Post Anesthesia Care Unit and Associate Professor of Anesthesiology, Thomas Jefferson University, Jefferson Medical College, Philadelphia, Pennsylvania

NIR HOFTMAN, MD
Associate Clinical Professor and Director of Thoracic Anesthesia, Department of Anesthesiology, University of California, Los Angeles, Los Angeles, California

TERESE T. HORLOCKER, MD
Professor of Anesthesiology and Orthopaedics, Department of Anesthesiology, Mayo Clinic, Rochester, Minnesota

BRIAN M. ILFELD, MD, MS (Clinical Investigation)
Associate Professor, In Residence Director of Clinical Research, Section of Regional Anesthesia and Acute Pain Medicine, Division of Pain Medicine, Department of Anesthesiology, University of California, San Diego, San Diego, California

TARA L. KNIZNER, MD
Resident, Department of Anesthesiology, University of Pittsburgh Medical Center, Pittsburgh, Pennsylvania

PILAR MERCADO, MD
Assistant Professor of Anesthesiology, Department of Anesthesiology, University of Illinois at Chicago, Chicago, Illinois

DENNIS P. PHILLIPS, DO
Associate Chief Resident, Department of Anesthesiology, University of Pittsburgh Medical Center, Pittsburgh, Pennsylvania

BRIAN SITES, MD
Associate Professor of Anesthesiology and Director of Orthopedic and Regional Anesthesia, Dartmouth-Hitchcock Medical Center, Dartmouth Medical School, Lebanon, New Hampshire

PAUL H. TING, MD
Staff Anesthesiologist, Albemarle Anesthesia, PLC, Martha Jefferson Hospital, Charlottesville, Virginia

EUGENE R. VISCUSI, MD
Director, Acute Pain Management and Associate Professor of Anesthesiology, Thomas Jefferson University, Jefferson Medical College, Philadelphia, Pennsylvania

GUY L. WEINBERG, MD
Professor of Anesthesiology, Department of Anesthesiology, University of Illinois
at Chicago; Jesse Brown Veterans Affairs Medical Center, Chicago, Illinois

BRIAN A. WILLIAMS, MD, MBA
Professor and Director, Division of Ambulatory Anesthesia, Department of
Anesthesiology, University of Pittsburgh School of Medicine, Pittsburgh, Pennsylvania

Contents

Ultrasound-guided regional anesthesia (UGRA) has increased in popularity over the past 5 years. This interest is reflected by the plethora of publications devoted to technique development, as well as randomized and controlled trials. Despite the excitement around ultrasonography, skeptics argue that there is a lack of evidence-based medicine to support the unequivocal adoption of UGRA as a "standard of care." This article summarizes and critically assesses current data comparing traditional approaches to localizing nerves with those that use ultrasound guidance. In addition, the potential benefits of UGRA that go beyond current information available from comparative studies are explored.

A single-injection peripheral nerve block using long-acting local anesthetic provides analgesia for 12 to 24 hours; however, many surgical procedures result in pain that lasts far longer. One relatively new option is a continuous peripheral nerve block (CPNB): local anesthetic is perfused via a perineural catheter directly adjacent to the peripheral nerve(s) supplying the surgical site, providing potent, site-specific analgesia. CPNB results in decreased pain, opioid requirements, opioid-related side effects, and sleep disturbances; in some cases, accelerating resumption of tolerated passive joint range-of-motion and increasing patient satisfaction. Ambulatory perineural infusion may be provided using a portable infusion pump, in some cases resulting in decreased hospitalization duration and related costs. Serious complications are rare, but may result in significant morbidity.

The use of regional anesthesia (RA) improves cost benefit (hospital-centered) and cost utility (patient-centered) over general anesthesia with volatile agents (GAVA), based upon research in outpatient populations. To make the cost savings a reality, the authors recommend: (1) avoidance of GAVA or at least volatile agents, (2) adopting published postanesthesia care unit (PACU)-bypass criteria conducive to RA, (3) maximizing PACU-bypass rates, and (4) utilizing a block induction area. Inpatient-based acute pain services are not uniform, which makes cost analyses and comparison between practices unreliable. Additional review and commentary address surgical site infections, cancer recurrence, blood transfusions, and chronic postsurgical pain.

Anesthesia is a sine qua non for most surgeries. Like any medical advance, progress in regional anesthesia has not come without its share of complications, including a spectrum extending from localized nerve injury to systemic cardiovascular toxicity and death. This article discusses the mechanisms and clinical presentation, prevention, treatment, and future trends of local anesthetic systemic toxicity. The adverse effects of lipid emulsion therapy are also included.

The incidence of neurologic damage after regional anesthesia is rare. However, this complication may have dramatic consequences for the patient because recovery may take several months. As nerve conduction studies and electromyography are the cornerstones of investigations in cases of postblock deficit, it is mandatory for the anesthesiologist performing regional anesthesia to have a basic understanding of these tests to discuss the cause with the surgeon and inform the patient about the prognosis.

Perioperative nerve injuries are recognized as a complication of regional anesthesia. Although rare, studies suggest the frequency of complications is increasing. Risk factors include neural, traumatic injury during needle or catheter placement, infection, and choice of local anesthetic solution. Neurologic injury due to pressure from improper patient positioning, tightly applied casts or surgical dressings, and surgical trauma are often attributed to regional anesthetic. Body habitus and preexisting neurologic dysfunction may also contribute. The safe conduct of regional anesthesia involves knowledge of patient, anesthetic, and surgical risk factors. Early diagnosis and treatment of reversible etiologies are critical to optimizing neurologic outcome.

Unintentional subdural injection during neuraxial anesthesia/analgesia continues to be a challenge for anesthesiologists. This unusual complication is often poorly recognized, with the diagnosis made in retrospect, or not at all. The clinical presentation of these regional blocks can be heterogeneous, ranging from restricted, patchy, or unilateral sensory blockade all the way to extensive and even life-threatening motor and autonomic nervous system depression. Prompt diagnosis using clinical algorithms and radiographic imaging is crucial for the early discontinuation of the offending catheter. Supportive care is mandatory in cases involving severe depression of consciousness, motor function, and/or sympathetic tone.

FORTHCOMING ISSUES

September 2011
Information Technology Applied to Anesthesiology
Kevin Tremper, MD, and
Sachin Kheterpal, MD, *Guest Editors*

December 2011
Vascular/Transplant Anesthesia
Rae M. Allain, MD, *Guest Editor*

RECENT ISSUES

March 2011
Quality of Anesthesia Care
Mark D. Neuman, MD, and
Elizabeth A. Martinez, MD, *Guest Editors*

December 2010
Perioperative Pharmacotherapy
Alan D. Kaye, MD, PhD, *Guest Editor*

September 2010
Current Topics in Anesthesia for Head and Neck Surgery
Joshua H. Atkins, MD, PhD,
and Jeff E. Mandel, MD, *Guest Editors*

RELATED INTEREST

Rheumatic Disease Clinics May 2008 (Volume 34, Issue 2)
Pain Mechanisms and Management in the Rheumatic Diseases
Mary-Ann Fitzcharles, MB, ChB, FRCP(C), *Guest Editor*

VISIT US ONLINE!
Access your subscription at:
www.theclinics.com

Foreword

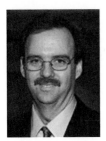

Lee A. Fleisher, MD
Consulting Editor

With the increasing emphasis on patient-oriented outcomes and delivery of cost-effective care, there has been a great deal of interest in the use of innovative methods to control acute postoperative pain. These include both novel medication management and the use of regional anesthetics. There is increasing evidence to suggest that these techniques can lead to earlier discharge with greater patient satisfaction related to control of pain symptoms. However, these are not without risks and costs. In this issue of *Anesthesiology Clinics*, the guest editors have solicited an outstanding collection of articles that highlight many of these issues including complications and the medical legal implications, enumeration of these techniques outside of the hospital, and the economic and practice management implications. In the clinical setting, the request to perform these techniques frequently comes from outside of the department and understanding these issues is critical. In the academic setting, our residents are excited to learn these techniques and to understand both the risks and the benefits.

To identify editors for this issue of *Clinics*, I reached out to two leaders of regional anesthesia from Canada. Dr Sugantha Ganapathy is currently Professor in the Department of Anesthesia and Perioperative Medicine at the University of Western Ontario and London Health Sciences Centre. She is Director of the Regional and Pain Research Division and has been an active investigator and leader in this area including being chair of the regional section of the Canadian Anesthesiologists Society. She has done an outstanding job in putting this issue together. She has been assisted by Dr Vincent Chan, Professor of Anesthesia at the University of Toronto. He has been an active leader in the field of regional anesthesia and is on the editorial boards of Anesthesia and Analgesia, and Regional Anesthesia and Pain Medicine. He is head of the regional anesthesia and pain program at University Health Network. He has been on the board of

doi:10.1016/j.anclin.2011.04.011
1932-2275/11/$
anesthesiology.theclinics.com

directors of the American Society of Regional Anesthesia and Pain Medicine since 1999. Together, they have assembled an outstanding issue.

Lee A. Fleisher, MD
University of Pennsylvania School of Medicine
3400 Spruce Street, Dulles 680
Philadelphia, PA 19104, USA

E-mail address:
lee.fleisher@uphs.upenn.edu

Preface

Regional Analgesia and Acute Pain Management: Major Leaps in Small Steps?

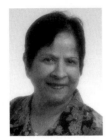 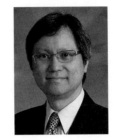

Sugantha Ganapathy, MBBS, DA, FRCA, FFARCS (I), FRCPC

Vincent Chan, MD, FRCPC

Guest Editors

Management of pain has evolved steadily over the past few years thanks to the knowledge derived from a large number of basic science and clinical research studies. While the management of chronic pain has utilized a significant amount of information from this research, acute pain management has benefited to a lesser extent. Our mainstay of therapy for acute pain remains opioid based, but we have realized that opioid drugs do a less-than-optimal job of relieving activity-associated pain in many acute scenarios. We have also realized the downside to using opioids as we see more and more patients with opioid tolerance, opioid-induced hyperalgesia, and immunosupression.

While brachial plexus block was performed through an open dissection almost a century ago, it is only in the last three decades that we have started the practice of regional nerve blockade for managing acute pain. Regional anesthesia provides excellent pain relief particularly for orthopedic surgery, and can significantly improve activity-associated pain and functional rehabilitation outcomes. The benefits of regional anesthesia are for patients, patients' families, as well as hospitals. For example, in the face of increasing economic restraints, regional anesthesia allows painful surgeries to be performed in outpatients by providing good quality pain relief at home. This can save hospital cost and utilization.

The use of continuous peripheral nerve block at home is a relatively new concept. With any such innovation, we inherit unique problems associated with adapting it into clinical practice. We have to make sure the block catheters are in perfect position in order to send patients home with them. The use of ultrasonograpy for regional anesthesia is gaining popularity, and there is growing evidence that ultrasound can improve nerve block accuracy. Drs Antonakakis, Ting, and Sites have provided an evidence-based comprehensive review of this topic for us in this issue of *Anesthesiology Clinics.* Dr Ilfeld tells us how to provide effective continuous perineural blockade in the hospital

Anesthesiology Clin 29 (2011) xiii–xiv
doi:10.1016/j.anclin.2011.04.012   anesthesiology.theclinics.com

and at home, and outlines the practical considerations for organizing a home care program. Drs Phillips, Knizner, and Williams provide an objective analysis of cost benefits and cost utility of regional anesthesia for acute pain management as compared to general anesthesia. The economic and practice management issues associated with acute pain management are discussed in detail. One of the major advances in local anesthetic toxicity research is the use of intralipid to counter local anesthetic-induced cardiovascular collapse. In this issue of *Anesthesiology Clinics*, Drs Mercado and Weinberg teach us how to prevent and manage local anesthetic systemic toxicity, and describe the scientific basis of using lipid emulsion.

Getting close to the nerves has potential for neurological injury. The pathophysiology and mechanism of injury is often difficult to define in the face of a postblock neurological deficit. Anesthesiologists are often ill prepared to defend or too ready to take the blame. In this issue we have Drs Borgeat and Aguirre, leading experts in this area, share with us their vast knowledge of evaluating postblock neurological deficits and effective treatment options. Dr Horlocker further reviews in detail the incidence and mechanisms of central and peripheral nerve injuries associated with regional anesthesia and acute pain management and provides recommendations to avoid them. Unintentional subdural injection, a complication of neuraxial anesthesia and analgesia, is thoroughly addressed by Dr Hoftman.

Yet not all postsurgical pain is amenable to some of these regional techniques. We also have patients with extraordinary requirements for pain management such as those with renal dysfunction and those receiving chronic opioid therapy, to mention but a few. In this issue Drs Gandhi, Heitz, and Viscusi give us pearls on how to manage such patients with multimodal analgesia.

While the regional blocks provide excellent analgesia for upper limb surgery, lower limb weakness and risk of fall associated with regional blocks are problematic. The development of local infiltration analgesia is a possible solution and the art of wound infusion of local anesthetics is described by Drs Ganapathy, Brookes, and Bourne.

Above all, we have come to realize the entity of chronic postsurgical pain. Can poorly managed acute pain result in chronic postsurgical pain? Dr de Kock tells us about prevention of such debilitating chronic pain following surgery.

This issue devoted to acute pain management aims to provide you with information that promotes high-caliber pain relief for your patients, both adults and children. We hope you enjoy reading this issue of *Anesthesiology Clinics*.

Sugantha Ganapathy, MBBS, DA, FRCA, FFARCS (I), FRCPC
Department of Anesthesiology and Perioperative Medicine
University of Western Ontario
B3213, London Health Sciences Centre, University Hospital
339 Windermere Road
London, Ontario N6A 5A5, Canada

Vincent Chan, MD, FRCPC
Department of Anesthesiology
University of Toronto
Toronto Western Hospital
399 Bathurst Street
Toronto, Ontario M5T 2S8, Canada

E-mail addresses:
Sugantha.Ganapathy@lhsc.on.ca (S. Ganapathy)
Vincent.Chan@uhn.on.ca (V. Chan)

Ultrasound-Guided Regional Anesthesia for Peripheral Nerve Blocks: An Evidence-Based Outcome Review

John G. Antonakakis, MD[a],*, Paul H. Ting, MD[b], Brian Sites, MD[c]

KEYWORD

• Ultrasonography • Regional • Anesthesia • Evidence
• Nerve blocks

Ultrasound-guided regional anesthesia (UGRA) has increased in popularity over the past 5 years. This interest is reflected by the plethora of publications devoted to technique development as well as randomized and controlled trials. The journal of the American Society of Regional Anesthesia and Pain Medicine (ASRA), *Regional Anesthesia and Pain Medicine*, has recently devoted a dedicated section to UGRA. Further evidence of the interest in ultrasonography by our community is the comprehensive coverage of UGRA at national and international meetings. Despite the excitement around ultrasound (US), skeptics argue that there is a lack of evidence-based medicine to support the unequivocal adoption of UGRA as a "standard of care." This article summarizes and critically assesses current data comparing traditional approaches to localizing nerves with those that use US guidance. In addition, the authors explore the potential benefits of UGRA that go beyond current information available from comparative studies.

CHARACTERIZING THE IDEAL REGIONAL ANESTHETIC

When comparing regional anesthesia with general anesthesia, general anesthesia is clearly the more popular choice for providing surgical anesthesia; this is especially

No funding or support was provided for this article.

The authors have no conflict of interest to declare.

[a] Department of Anesthesiology, Portsmouth Regional Hospital, 333 Borthwick Avenue, Portsmouth, NH 03801, USA

[b] Department of Anesthesiology, Albemarle Anesthesia, PLC, Martha Jefferson Hospital, 459 Locust Avenue, Charlottesville, VA 22902, USA

[c] Department of Anesthesiology, Dartmouth-Hitchcock Medical Center, Dartmouth Medical School, One Medical Center Drive, Lebanon, NH 03756, USA

* Corresponding author. 29 Chisholm Farm Drive, Stratham, NH 03885.

E-mail address: jantonakakis@gmail.com

Anesthesiology Clin 29 (2011) 179–191

doi:10.1016/j.anclin.2011.04.008

1932-2275/11/$ – see front matter © 2011 Published by Elsevier Inc.

anesthesiology.theclinics.com

true in many smaller community hospitals. General anesthesia is reproducible, nearly painless, is easy to perform, enjoys a rapid onset, and has a near 100% success rate. In addition, general anesthesia is safer than it has ever been as a result of current state-of-the-art advances in monitoring, drug development, and airway devices. However, regional anesthesia has indisputable advantages in anesthesia practice. Regional anesthesia provides superior pain control, decreases opioid-related morbidity, and decreases hospital admissions.[1,2] Such attributes may serve to improve meaningful long-term outcomes.[3] Although these benefits are generally agreed upon, the mechanism by which we can generate a successful block, to realize such benefits, is subject to debate. Specifically, is US "better" than traditional landmark techniques? To answer this question, we must first define the outcome variables that characterize "better." The following list summarizes important outcome variables:

1. Performed quickly and easily by most anesthesiologists
2. Facilitates faster onset of block
3. Provides for a reliable and predictable quality block with appropriate duration
4. Minimal patient discomfort
5. Reduction in dose of local anesthetic required
6. Improved safety profile
7. Easy to teach with objective end points
8. Allows for the expansion of the practice of regional anesthesia.

Although few may argue with the points in this list, whether UGRA can provide all of these advantages over traditional techniques is unclear. We should now look at what the existing literature can tell us, so as to critically assess these important end points of regional anesthesia. The majority of the randomized controlled trials (RCTs) performed to date focus on upper extremity and lower extremity nerve blocks. For the purposes of this review, the authors sought to review RCTs that specifically compared US alone with traditional landmark techniques. In addition, the focus is predominately on studies that have a clearly defined specific end point as the primary outcome and are adequately powered to detect that primary outcome.

PERFORMANCE TIME

Performance time, or the time necessary to perform the block, is an important quality measure when practicing regional anesthesia. Nineteen RCTs that recorded performance time were identified.[4–22] In 6 of these RCTs, it was the primary outcome measured.[5,13,18–21] The definition of performance time varied in different studies. For US-guided nerve blocks, 2 common definitions of performance time were: (1) the time interval between needle puncture to the end of local anesthetic injection or needle removal, therefore excluding the US scanning time; or (2) the time interval between US transducer placement on the patient to the end of local anesthetic injection or needle removal. For landmark nerve blocks a common definition for performance time was the time from needle placement to the end of local anesthetic injection or needle removal. In 11 of the 19 RCTs,[7–13,18,20–22] US had a statistically significant advantage in minimizing the performance time over conventional landmark techniques, whereas 5 RCTs[4–6,14,19] demonstrated no difference. Three RCTs[15–17] involving ankle blocks in volunteers favored the landmark approach. It is important to note that the US scanning and image acquisition times were not included in the 5 RCTs[4,7,13,14,22] that either favored the use of US or showed no difference in performance time. On the contrary, in these same 5 RCTs the landmark groups did not include the time consumed in palpating and/or drawing out the superficial landmarks. Nevertheless, the literature overall appears to support the use of US in minimizing performance time.

ONSET TIME

Most RCTs defined onset time as the time interval from the injection of local anesthetic and removal of the needle to a complete sensory block. Similar to performance time, onset time is an important quality measure when performing regional anesthesia. The authors identified 17 RCTs in which onset time was clearly defined and measured.[4-14,17,23-27] Fourteen RCTs favored the use of US in minimizing the onset time.[4,6,8-13,17,23-27] In 3 RCTs[5,7,14] there was no statistical difference in onset time between the US group and the traditional landmark groups. When looking at onset time as the primary outcome variable, 5 of 7 of RCTs favored the use of US in minimizing the onset time,[6,9,24-26] while in 2 RCTs[5,7] there was no statistical difference between US and landmark techniques. It must be noted that in 2 of the frequently quoted RCTs[24,25] favoring the use of US in minimizing onset time, onset time was the primary outcome variable measured; however, a power analysis was not performed. Caution must be exercised when interpreting these results.[28] Nevertheless, US appears to decrease the overall onset time by 2 to 12 minutes when performing a nerve block,[4-14,23-27] perhaps because US allows for closer needle approximation and local anesthetic distribution to the target nerves.

It has been argued that the improvement in onset time, although statistically significant, may perhaps be clinically irrelevant.[29] Similar to performance time, the authors believe that any time saved is valuable from a perspective of quality improvement. The clinical significance of decreasing onset time, decreasing performance time, and therefore decreasing surgical readiness from regional anesthesia depends on the characteristics of the individual practice. A busy practice setting, with rapid and frequent room turnover, would likely benefit most as operating room throughput is maximized. In addition, the ability to decrease onset time and performance time will facilitate the anesthesiologist in making a timely decision regarding the need to provide block supplement or convert to general anesthesia.

QUALITY

The definition of the quality of a nerve block varies between different RCTs. Most RCTs define the success or the quality of a nerve block as a complete sensory nerve block in all nerve territories examined by a predefined time period, that is, 20 to 30 minutes. However, when a nerve block is used as the surgical anesthetic, other definitions of quality include the need for analgesic supplementation or conversion to general anesthesia. Of importance, a nerve block that does not achieve a complete sensory block within a predefined time frame does not always lead to the need for supplemental analgesics or conversions to general anesthesia; this is because a nerve block may have achieved surgical conditions at a point beyond the 20 to 30 minutes, which is the usual time frame for the current studies. It can be argued that the need for conversion from a regional anesthetic to a general anesthetic is a more objective measure of the quality of a nerve block than relying on the more subjective sensory loss assessment.

The authors identified 25 RCTs in which the quality or efficacy of a nerve block was assessed.[4-23,26,27,30-32] Assessments were based on one or more of the following: complete sensory block at a predefined time interval, the need for supplemental local or systemic analgesics, conversion to general anesthesia, or the quality of postoperative analgesia. Overall, 15 of the 25 RCTs showed some benefit to the use of US over landmark techniques,[6,8,10,11,14–17,21–23,27,30–32] whereas 10 studies did not find any difference in the quality of nerve block regardless of technique.[4,5,7,9,12,13,18–20,26] In no RCTs was the quality of a block superior in the landmark technique as compared with a US-guided technique. Seventeen[4–12,18–21,23,26,27,32] of the 25 RCTs specifically measured the conversion from regional anesthesia to general anesthesia because of a failed surgical block. On critical evaluation of these data, 13 of the 17 RCTs[4–10,12,18–20,26,27] showed no statistical difference between US and a landmark technique, while 4 of the 17 RCTs[11,21,23,32] supported the use of US. One may wonder why the results comparing US and landmark techniques are equivocal when "success" is measured by the conversion of regional anesthesia to general anesthesia. It is important to be aware that most RCTs are not powered to detect this difference, and caution must be exercised when interpreting these results.[28] In fact, the quality assessment of a nerve bock serving as the primary outcome occurred in 11 of the 25 RCTs.[6,8,10,11,15–17,22,27,31,32] However, in only 1 of these 11 RCTs was "failed surgical blocks" the quality measure of interest.[11] The remaining 10 RCTs assessed "complete sensory block" and not "failed surgical blocks." The conversion of regional anesthesia to surgical anesthesia is a more objective measure of block quality and success than is assessing loss of sensation. When assessing the "quality" of a peripheral nerve block as defined by the conversion of regional anesthesia to general anesthesia, larger and adequately powered RCTs are needed to perhaps detect a statistical difference between US and landmark techniques.

PATIENT SAFETY

Compared with conventional landmark techniques, US offers anesthesia providers the distinct ability to visualize neural structures, surrounding tissues, the needle, and the correct spread of local anesthetic. Whether these advantages translate to improved patient safety is subject to debate.[33,34] Complications or side effects of interest included neurologic injury, local anesthetic systemic toxicity, pneumothorax, and hemidiaphragmatic paresis (HDP). US may allow the anesthesiologist to avoid vascular trauma, nerve trauma, and intravascular injection.

Of the RCTs directly comparing US alone with traditional landmark techniques, 3 RCTs[5,8,27] were identified in which US resulted in a statistically significant reduction in unintended paresthesias during block placement. The authors also identified 4 RCTs in which US resulted in a decrease in the incidence of vascular puncture compared with landmark techniques.[5,10,19,21] Liu and colleagues,[12] studying adverse events as the primary outcome during axillary blocks, reported a decrease in the overall incidence of paresthesia, vessel puncture, and subcutaneous hematoma by using US. In a prospective observational study, Borgeat and colleagues[35] demonstrated that postoperative neurologic symptoms are common after interscalene nerve blocks and shoulder surgery. Using traditional landmark techniques they reported an incidence of 14% at 10 days and 0.2% at 9 months. Liu and colleagues,[4] using neurologic symptoms as the primary outcome and powered to detect a fourfold decrease (16%–4%) with the use of US, did not show a statistically significant difference in outcome between US and landmark techniques. It must be noted that Liu and colleagues used large volumes of local anesthetic (45–55 mL for <50 kg and 55–65 mL for >50 kg) in both groups. Given that local anesthetics are to some degree neurotoxic and that US has proven to reduce the volume of local anesthetic required for successful nerve blockade, it is unknown if reducing the volume of local anesthetic will decrease the incidence of postoperative neurologic symptoms.

Peripheral nerve injury after regional anesthesia is multifactorial.[34] Factors involved include anesthetic risk factors as well as surgical and patient risk factors. Anesthetic risk factors involved in perioperative nerve injury include mechanical trauma, neural ischemia, and local anesthetic neurotoxicity. By directly visualizing key structures (needle, nerve, and local anesthetic), US has potential to modify risk factors such as mechanical nerve injury. In addition, local anesthetic neurotoxicity may be decreased by the use of smaller volumes of local anesthetic. The possibility of neural ischemia may be additionally reduced if compressive neuropathies from hematoma formation can be avoided. US will not, however, have any direct impact on patient risk factors such as sex, increasing age, elevated body mass index, preexisting nerve damage, or surgical risk factors.[34] US may have the ability to identify sonopathology such as neuritis, anatomic variation, and peripheral nerve tumors allowing modification or abortion of the block plan.[36–38] Overall, limited literature directly comparing UGRA to traditional landmark techniques would suggest that UGRA neither increases nor decreases short-term or long-term peripheral nerve injury. This result is in agreement with a large prospective audit of more than 7000 peripheral nerve blocks in which unintended paresthesia during block placement and block-related late neurologic injury did not differ between UGRA and landmark techniques.[39]

Local anesthetic systemic toxicity may occur from a direct intravascular injection or by systemic absorption. US has the potential to decrease the rate of local anesthetic toxicity by avoiding intravascular injections and reducing local anesthetic volumes. Multiple investigators have demonstrated that US allows for effective nerve blockade with smaller volumes of local anesthetic.[14–17,39,40] US allows for precise needle to nerve proximity, and therefore avoids using "volume" as a vehicle for effective nerve blockade. For example, it is routine for the authors to use 5 to 10 mL of local anesthetic to provide an effective interscalene brachial plexus nerve block, not the 45 to 65 mL used in the study by Liu and colleagues.[4]

It is debatable whether an HDP should be considered a "complication" as opposed to a "side effect" of interscalene nerve blocks, because HDP has traditionally been reported to have a 100% incidence with interscalene nerve blocks. Nevertheless, preliminary data would suggest that US might reduce the incidence of HDP with smaller volumes of local anesthetic.[41,42] Riazi and colleagues[41] demonstrated an approximately 55% reduction in the incidence of diaphragmatic paralysis when low volumes (5 mL) of local anesthetic was injected versus standard volumes (20 mL) without difference in pain scores, sleep quality, or morphine consumption up to 24 hours. In addition, patients with phrenic nerve palsy in the low-volume group had significantly better preservation of lung function than the high-volume group.[42] Although these results are promising, a 50% incidence of HDP with low-volume US-guided nerve blocks is still clinically significant and would possibly preclude this block in a patient with critically compromised pulmonary function. However, this study allows us to make better-informed risk benefit decisions in patients with mild and perhaps moderate compromise in pulmonary function. In an RCT, Renes and colleagues[30] compared the incidence of diaphragmatic paresis between US-guided interscalene nerve blocks and traditional nerve stimulator landmark techniques. Diaphragmatic paresis occurred in 2 of 15 (14.3%) patients in the US group and 14 of 15 (93.3%) patients in the nerve stimulator (NS) group (P<.0001). Of importance, the 2 patients in the US group with diaphragmatic paresis had complete recovery of diaphragm movement and ventilatory function by 180 min. These investigators used 10 mL of 0.75% ropivacaine and injected posterior and lateral to the C7 nerve root. In a similar study Renes and colleagues[43] also examined the incidence of diaphragmatic paresis during a supraclavicular nerve block, and demonstrated a 50%

incidence of HDP during an NS technique and 0% incidence during a US technique. Spirometric function was preserved in the US group while it was significantly reduced in the landmark group. To achieve these results the investigators used 20 mL of 0.75% ropivacaine while injecting in a careful manner caudal and posterolateral to the brachial plexus. Despite these promising results for both interscalene and supraclavicular blocks, they should be considered preliminary data because of the small number of patients. These two studies are unique in the US literature in that the investigators intimately describe the morphology of spread of local anesthetics that generated their results. To accurately study, verify, and translate research findings into routine practice, the regional anesthesia community needs to be able to consistently reproduce the desired spread of local anesthetics. In the era of nerve stimulation, the defined motor response was always sought and well appreciated; now, it is the "correct" perineural spread. This "correctness" must be explicitly defined. Most studies lack detailed explanations of "bad" versus "good" spreads.[44]

A pneumothorax is a serious complication of regional anesthesia, which may occur during the performance of a paravertebral, infraclavicular, or supraclavicular nerve block. Pneumothorax with supraclavicular nerve blocks has traditionally been a real concern with landmark-based techniques. Through direct visualization, US has the potential to eliminate this devastating complication. US has repopularized supraclavicular nerve blocks in recent years. In a series of 500 patients undergoing US supraclavicular nerve blocks, Perlas and colleagues[45] did not report a single incidence of a pneumothorax. Although 500 patients is a relatively small number on which to base any firm conclusion on the safety of preventing a pneumothorax with UGRA, a recent query of the Dartmouth Hitchcock Medical Center regional anesthesia database resulted in 1433 US-guided supraclavicular nerve blocks performed with trainees without a single pneumothorax being encountered.

One must acknowledge that although US has the potential to avoid complications of mechanical nerve injury, intravascular injections, and pneumothorax, case reports of these events do occur even with the use of US.[46–49] Such outcomes stem primarily from the training and experience of the anesthesiologist using US technology. It is the authors' observational experience that novices inexperienced with US-guided nerve blocks misinterpret US images. In addition, the appropriate skill set of maintaining simultaneous visualization of the nerves, needle, and local anesthetic injection takes time and practice to develop. Sites and colleagues[50] demonstrated that failure to visualize the needle during advancement occurred in up to 43% of novices (<10 US-guided blocks). As experience with UGRA grows and appropriate training occurs through residency programs as well as training pathways for anesthesiologists in practice, UGRA has the potential in experienced hands to decrease and possibly eliminate the incidence of these avoidable complications.

LIMITATIONS OF THE CURRENT RCTS

It appears from the data presented that US decreases the amount of local anesthetic, shortens the onset time, and quickens the performance time. It may also perhaps improve the efficacy of the block. However, some of the current RCTs do not fairly compare landmark with US techniques. For example, Kapral and colleagues[23] showed that US improved the quality of an interscalene nerve block compared with a traditional landmark technique. In their study, US allowed for a successful surgical anesthetic in 98.8% of patients while landmark with nerve stimulation had a 91.3% success rate ($P<.01$). However, Kapral and colleagues used a hand and forearm motor response in the NS group and not a deltoid/bicep response, which would have been the preferred motor response.[51,52] Accepting a bicep/deltoid response may have altered their final results. To draw a meaningful conclusion, future studies should use the best NS response for the landmark/NS groups.[51,53]

For most practitioners, nerve stimulation is a single injection technique. A nerve is localized by obtaining the appropriate motor response and the local anesthetic is deposited in one location. US, on the other hand, is a multi-injection technique, as the needle may be repositioned several times to obtain the appropriate spread of local anesthetic. Therefore, it has been suggested that to fairly compare US with nerve stimulation, a multi-injection NS group should be compared with a US group.[50] For example, Perlas and colleagues[6] demonstrated a higher success rate (defined by loss of sensation of the tibial and common peroneal nerve at 30 minutes) during popliteal sciatic nerve blocks when using a pure US-guided technique compared with a landmark technique for foot and ankle surgery. In the US technique, the needle was positioned as needed to guide the appropriate spread of local anesthetic. However, in the landmark technique a single injection was performed after obtaining any foot or toe response. This study has been criticized because the appropriate motor response (a tibial nerve response and specifically foot inversion) was not elicited. However, would a double stimulation technique by obtaining a tibial nerve and common peroneal nerve have altered their results? Danelli and colleagues[9] performed a similar study, comparing US with a double stimulation landmark technique for foot and ankle surgery. Specifically, the landmark group elicited a common peroneal and tibial nerve motor response at 0.4 mA. However, Danelli and colleagues were not able to detect a statistical difference between groups with respect to a complete sensory and motor block at 30 minutes or a difference in the conversion to general anesthesia. Although these results conflict with those of Perlas and colleagues, the authors believe that a double stimulation technique is concerning on several fronts. First, most anesthesiologists using US will reposition the needle only if local anesthetic is not covering the target structure. In a double stimulation technique, the second injection may be completely unnecessary. Further, the significant false-negative rate of NS must be considered,[54,55] especially in the setting of a previous bolus of local anesthetic. Even if US-guided nerve blocks are equivocal to a multistimulation landmark technique, US has a distinct advantage of allowing for real-time visualization of the needle and correct spread of local anesthetic while potentially avoiding mechanical nerve trauma.

RCTs comparing US with landmark techniques are usually performed at medical centers with well-organized and successful regional anesthesia programs. Experts in regional anesthesia are usually performing or at least supervising novices performing these nerve blocks. Therefore, the results seen in RCTs may not reflect what occurs in the larger community. The proficient conduct of UGRA requires a skill set that is unique from traditional landmark techniques, including the mastering of 2-dimensional image interpretation. This difference must be considered when interpreting the results of any clinical trials. Operator bias, with respect to both techniques, is a real and unavoidable limitation. Current and past studies reveal essentially no objective information regarding the training and proficiency of the operators. If the results of an adequately powered trial reveal "no difference" between US versus nerve stimulation, is it because the operators were really experts only in nerve stimulation? In fact, one could argue that the results should be interpreted as a "win" for US because equivalence was demonstrated despite the fact that the operators were not as equally skilled in both techniques. This situation is likely to be a common one, as many "expert" groups have been performing UGRA for 5 years or less, whereas the experience with nerve stimulation goes back to the early 1990s. It should be noted that operator bias can be argued from both sides of the aisle, with many emerging research groups only expert in US and with little NS experience.

EDUCATING THE ANESTHESIOLOGIST IN ULTRASOUND-GUIDED REGIONAL ANESTHESIA

No RCTs have characterized the learning curves and early success rates for US-guided regional anesthesia versus traditional landmark-based regional anesthesia. For a community-based anesthesiologist interested in offering regional anesthesia to his or her patients, would attending a workshop in either US-guided regional anesthesia or traditional landmark-based regional anesthesia lead to differing success? It is the authors' anecdotal experience with teaching residents and practicing anesthesiologists in regional anesthesia that US may decrease the learning curve and provide early success. The idea of sonographically objectifying the steps of a nerve block allows needle and injection corrections based on defined goals rather than assumptions of unconfirmed anatomy. These benefits are especially attractive to the supervisor of the novice. With respect to the popular supraclavicular block, if a novice follows a traditional NS approach and advances the needle, and no twitch occurs, what are the next steps? What does the supervisor recommend? The authors' suspicion is that the recommendations would be quite variable. "Fanning" the needle to contact the first rib as described by leading textbooks[56] would unlikely be championed by the novice or supervisor. However, using the in-plane US approach, the novice can see that the needle is lateral to the brachial plexus (as an example) and thus the operator objectively decides to redirect the needle closer to the subclavian artery. Using this supraclavicular example, it makes sense that there are suggestions in the literature supporting the notion that it is easier to guide a novice through a successful US-guided nerve block than through a landmark-based technique with nerve stimulations. Mariano and colleagues,[18,19,21] assessing trainees placing popliteal sciatic, femoral, and infraclavicular catheters, suggested that trainees had relative ease in placing peripheral nerve catheters using US compared with landmark and NS-based techniques. When performing infraclavicular catheters, trainees successfully placed 14 of 20 nerve catheters using nerve stimulation. However using US, all 20 catheters were successfully placed by trainees ($P<.01$).[21]

Sites and colleagues[50] characterized the behavior of novice residents in training during a dedicated 1-month rotation in US-guided regional anesthesia. The two most common errors consisted of failure to visualize the needle before advancement and unintentional probe movement. Other quality-compromising behaviors identified in novices were: (1) failure to recognize the maldistribution of local anesthesia, (2) failure to recognize an intramuscular location of the needle tip before injection, (3) fatigue, (4) failure to correctly correlate the sidedness of the patient with the sidedness of the US image, and (5) poor choice of needle-insertion site and angle with respect to the probe preventing accurate needle visualization. However, both speed and accuracy improved throughout the rotation. All residents performed at least 66 nerve blocks, with an overall success rate of 93.6% and 4 complications.

In 2009 the American Society of Regional Anesthesia in a conjoint effort with the European Society of Regional Anesthesia established new guidelines and a curriculum for US-guided regional anesthesia.[57] The purpose of creating of this document was to define the scope of practice related to UGRA and to recommend practice pathways useful in gaining clinical competency. The guidelines specifically define the core competencies and skill sets associated with UGRA and suggest 10 common tasks to be followed when performing an US-guided nerve block. In addition, the guidelines suggest a residency-based training pathway as well as a training practice pathway for postgraduate anesthesiologists.

EXPANDING THE BENEFITS OF REGIONAL ANESTHESIA VIA ULTRASOUND TECHNOLOGY

In the past, outcomes from anesthesia included whether a patient survived surgery and was discharged from the hospital.[3] Important modern-day outcomes positively influenced by the application of regional anesthesia include, but are not limited to, postoperative analgesia, nausea and vomiting, postoperative ileus formation, urinary retention, unplanned hospital admissions, and patient satisfaction.[1,2] Long-term outcomes that may be positively influenced by regional anesthesia include the reduction in chronic pain syndromes and the prevention of cancer recurrence.[3,58] Current RCTs consistently demonstrate that block onset and patient readiness for surgery is faster when US techniques are used as compared with traditional landmark techniques. In a busy practice setting with rapid turnover, surgical readiness from regional anesthesia is critical. Achieving surgical readiness quickly may affect whether these benefits of regional anesthesia are even offered to patients. The authors support the notion that any time saving is good, even if the reality is that it is less than 5 minutes.

There is currently a paucity of RCTs adequately powered to determine whether US improves the quality and success of peripheral nerve block as defined by the conversion to general anesthesia from regional anesthesia. Most studies assess this end point as a secondary outcome. Based on the current evidence, it is probably safe to conclude that US may not improve the success of a peripheral nerve block as defined by the conversion of regional anesthesia to general anesthesia. However, one must remember that in RCTs, experts are performing both US and landmark techniques, and success rates in RCTs may not translate to the success rate of an individual practitioner. For the sake of argument, let us assume that US and nerve stimulation are equivalent in terms of the generation of surgical anesthesia. Given that the "ultrasound" revolution has unequivocally expanded the use of regional anesthesia, one would have to accept that US is responsible for an improvement in meaningful outcomes such as improved postoperative analgesia, and decreased postoperative nausea/vomiting, ileus formation, urinary retention, unexpected hospital admissions, and opioid consumption, as well as overall improvement in patient satisfaction. Therefore, the question should not be "is ultrasound better?" but rather "can US improve meaningful perioperative outcomes by increasing the application of regional anesthesia?" It is the authors' contention that regional anesthesia is now practiced by individuals who originally rejected regional techniques when they were based on anatomic assumptions without image guidance.

SUMMARY

US technology has been a significant advancement in the practice of regional anesthesia, with growing evidence to support its use. When compared with other forms of nerve localization, the data support its use in decreasing performance time and onset time, and therefore decreasing the time for surgical readiness from regional anesthesia. The quality of peripheral nerve blocks also appears to favor UGRA. There are insufficient data to declare that UGRA improves overall block success as defined by the conversion of regional anesthesia to general anesthesia. However, the authors believe that any surrogate to block success that improves the quality of a block as well as decreases the time to surgical readiness from regional anesthesia is clinically important, because these surrogates factor into the decision making of whether regional anesthesia is offered to patients in the first place. Therefore if US, through its proven surrogate measures of block success, is able to expand the application of regional anesthesia, then arguably UGRA will have proven clinical advantages over other methods of nerve localization. Although it is difficult to prove that UGRA can improve patient safety, by allowing for the use of smaller volumes of local anesthetic as well as the real-time interaction of the needle, the nerve, and the local anesthetic, US may decrease the risk of a pneumothorax or hemidiaphragmatic paresis, as well as local anesthetic systemic and neuronal toxicity. Future RCTs are needed with larger numbers of patients powered to detect a difference in block success as defined by the conversion of regional anesthesia to general anesthesia. These RCTs should objectify and consistently reproduce the correct perineural spread of local anesthetic to accurately study, verify, and translate research findings into routine practice. Finally, it must be emphasized that US is a powerful tool for nerve localization, and sufficient anatomic knowledge, training, and judgment are essential for the safe practice of UGRA.

REFERENCES

1. Hadzic A, Williams BA, Karaca PE, et al. For outpatient rotator cuff surgery, nerve block anesthesia provides superior same-day recovery over general anesthesia. Anesthesiology 2005;102:1001–7.
2. Brown A, Weiss R, Greenberg C, et al. Interscalene block for shoulder arthroscopy: comparison with general anesthesia. Arthroscopy 1993;9:295–300.
3. Sessler DI. Long-term consequences of anesthetic management. Anesthesiology 2009;111:1–4.
4. Liu SS, Zayas VM, Gordon MA, et al. A prospective, randomized, controlled trial comparing ultrasound versus nerve stimulator guidance for interscalene block for ambulatory shoulder surgery for postoperative neurologic symptoms. Anesth Analg 2009;109:265–71.
5. Sauter AR, Dodgson MS, Stubhaug A, et al. Electrical nerve stimulation or ultrasound guidance for lateral sagittal infraclavicular blocks: a randomized, controlled, observer blinded comparison study. Anesth Analg 2008;106:1910–5.
6. Perlas A, Brull R, Chan VW, et al. Ultrasound guidance improves the success of sciatic nerve block at the popliteal fossa. Reg Anesth Pain Med 2008;33:259–65.
7. Taboada M, Rodríguez J, Amor M, et al. Is ultrasound guidance superior to conventional nerve stimulation for coracoid infraclavicular brachial plexus? Reg Anesth Pain Med 2009;34:357–60.
8. Brull R, Lupu M, Perlas A, et al. Compared with dual nerve stimulation, ultrasound guidance shortens the time for infraclavicular block performance. Can J Anaesth 2009;56:812–8.
9. Danelli G, Fanelli A, Ghisi D, et al. Ultrasound vs nerve stimulation multiple injection technique for posterior popliteal sciatic nerve block. Anaesthesia 2009;64:638–42.
10. Chan VW, Perlas A, McCartney CJ, et al. Ultrasound guidance improves success rate of axillary brachial plexus block. Can J Anaesth 2007;54:176–82.
11. Sites BD, Beach ML, Spence BC, et al. Ultrasound guidance improves the success rate of a perivascular axillary plexus block. Acta Anaesthesiol Scand 2006;50:678–84.
12. Liu FC, Liou JT, Tsai YF, et al. Efficacy of ultrasound-guided axillary brachial plexus block: a comparative study with nerve stimulator-guided method. Chang Gung Med J 2005;28:396–402.

13. Macaire P, Singelyn F, Narchi P, et al. Ultrasound- or nerve stimulation-guided wrist blocks for carpal tunnel release: a randomized prospective comparative study. Reg Anesth Pain Med 2008;33:363–8.
14. van Geffen GJ, van den Broek E, Braak GJ, et al. A prospective randomised controlled trial of ultrasound guided versus nerve stimulation guided distal sciatic nerve block at the popliteal fossa. Anaesth Intensive Care 2009;37:32–7.
15. Redborg KE, Antonakakis JG, Beach ML, et al. Ultrasound improves the success rate of a tibial nerve block at the ankle. Reg Anesth Pain Med 2009;34:256–60.
16. Redborg KE, Sites BD, Chinn CD, et al. Ultrasound improves the success rate of a sural nerve block at the ankle. Reg Anesth Pain Med 2009;34:24–8.
17. Antonakakis JG, Scalzo DC, Jorgenson AS, et al. Ultrasound does not improve the success rate of a deep peroneal nerve block at the ankle. Reg Anesth Pain Med 2010;35:217–21.
18. Mariano ER, Cheng GS, Choy LP, et al. Electrical stimulation versus ultrasound guidance for popliteal-sciatic perineural catheter insertion: a randomized control trial. Reg Anesth Pain Med 2009;34:480–5.
19. Mariano ER, Loland VJ, Sandhu NS, et al. Ultrasound guidance versus electrical stimulation for femoral perineural catheter insertion. J Ultrasound Med 2009;28:1453–60.
20. Mariano ER, Loland VJ, Sandhu NS, et al. A trainee-based randomized comparison of stimulating interscalene perineural catheters with a new technique using ultrasound guidance alone. J Ultrasound Med 2010;29:329–36.
21. Mariano ER, Loland VJ, Bellars RH, et al. Ultrasound guidance versus electrical stimulation for infraclavicular brachial plexus perineural catheter insertion. J Ultrasound Med 2009;28:1211–8.
22. Fredrickson MJ, Ball CM, Dalgleish AJ. A prospective randomized comparison of ultrasound guidance versus neurostimulation for interscalene catheter placement. Reg Anesth Pain Med 2009;34:590–4.
23. Kapral S, Greher M, Huber G, et al. Ultrasonographic guidance improves the success rate of interscalene brachial plexus blockade. Reg Anesth Pain Med 2008;33:253–8.
24. Marhofer P, Schrögendorfer K, Koinig H, et al. Ultrasonographic guidance improves sensory block and onset time of three-in-one blocks. Anesth Analg 1997;85:854–7.
25. Marhofer P, Schrögendorfer K, Wallner T, et al. Ultrasonographic guidance reduces the amount of local anesthetic for 3-in-1 blocks. Reg Anesth Pain Med 1998;23:584–8.
26. Casati A, Danelli G, Baciarello M, et al. A prospective, randomized comparison between ultrasound and nerve stimulation guidance for multiple injection axillary brachial plexus block. Anesthesiology 2007;106:992–6.
27. Soeding PE, Sha S, Royse CE, et al. A randomized trial of ultrasound-guided brachial plexus anaesthesia in upper limb surgery. Anaesth Intensive Care 2005;33:719–25.
28. Mariano ER, Ilfeld BM, Neal JM. "Going fishing"—the practice of reporting secondary outcomes as separate studies. Reg Anesth Pain Med 2007;32:183–5.
29. Neal JM, Brull R, Chan VW, et al. The ASRA evidence-based medicine assessment of ultrasound-guided regional anesthesia and pain medicine: executive summary. Reg Anesth Pain Med 2010;35:S1–9.
30. Renes SH, Rettig HC, Gielen MJ, et al. Ultrasound-guided low-dose interscalene brachial plexus block reduces the incidence of hemidiaphragmatic paresis. Reg Anesth Pain Med 2009;34:498–502.

31. Dolan J, Williams A, Murney E, et al. Ultrasound guided fascia iliaca block: a comparison with the loss of resistance technique. Reg Anesth Pain Med 2008;33:526–31.
32. Dhir S, Ganapathy S. Comparative evaluation of ultrasound-guided continuous infraclavicular brachial plexus block with stimulating catheter and traditional technique: a prospective-randomized trial. Acta Anaesthesiol Scand 2008;52:1158–66.
33. Neal JM. Ultrasound-guided regional anesthesia and patient safety: an evidence-based analysis. Reg Anesth Pain Med 2010;35:S59–67.
34. Hebl JR. Ultrasound-guided regional anesthesia and the prevention of neurologic injury: fact or fiction? Anesthesiology 2008;108:186–8.
35. Borgeat A, Ekatodramis G, Kalberer F, et al. Acute and nonacute complications associated with interscalene block and shoulder surgery: a prospective study. Anesthesiology 2001;95:875–80.
36. Sites BD, Macfarlane AJ, Sites VR, et al. Clinical sonopathology for the regional anesthesiologist part 1: vascular and neural. Reg Anesth Pain Med 2010;35:272–80.
37. Sites BD, Macfarlane AJ, Sites VR, et al. Clinical sonopathology for the regional anesthesiologist: part 2: bone, viscera, subcutaneous tissue, and foreign bodies. Reg Anesth Pain Med 2010;35:281–9.
38. Sites BD, Spence BC, Gallagher JD, et al. On the edge of the ultrasound screen: regional anesthesiologists diagnosing nonneural pathology. Reg Anesth Pain Med 2006;31:555–62.
39. Barrington MJ, Watts SA, Gledhill SR, et al. Preliminary results of the Australasian Regional Anaesthesia Collaboration: a prospective audit of more than 7000 peripheral nerve and plexus blocks for neurologic and other complications. Reg Anesth Pain Med 2009;34:534–41.
40. Casati A, Baciarello M, Di Cianni S, et al. Effects of ultrasound guidance on the minimum effective anaesthetic volume required to block the femoral nerve. Br J Anaesth 2007;98:823–7.
41. Riazi S, Carmichael N, Awad I, et al. Effect of local anesthetic volume (20 vs. 5 ml) on the efficacy and respiratory consequences of ultrasound-guided interscalene brachial plexus block. Br J Anaesth 2008;101:549–56.
42. McCartney CJL, Carmichael NM, Riazi S, et al. Reply: does low-volume interscalene block attenuate the severity of diaphragmatic paresis? Br J Anaesth 2009;102:142.
43. Renes SH, Spoormans HH, Gielen MJ, et al. Hemidiaphragmatic paresis can be avoided in ultrasound-guided supraclavicular brachial plexus block. Reg Anesth Pain Med 2009;34:595–9.
44. Sites BD, Neal JM, Chan V. Ultrasound in regional anesthesia: where should the "focus" be set? Reg Anesth Pain Med 2009;34:531–3.
45. Perlas A, Lobo G, Lo N, et al. Ultrasound-guided supraclavicular block: outcome of 510 consecutive cases. Reg Anesth Pain Med 2009;34:171–6.
46. Gnaho A, Eyrieux S, Gentili ME. Cardiac arrest during an ultrasound-guided sciatic nerve block combined with nerve stimulation. Reg Anesth Pain Med 2009;34:278.
47. Zetlaoui RJ, Labbe JP, Benhamou D. Ultrasound guidance for axillary plexus block does not prevent intravascular injection. Anesthesiology 2008;108:761.
48. Bryan NA, Swenson JD, Greis PE, et al. Indwelling interscalene catheter use in an outpatient setting for shoulder surgery: technique, efficacy, and complications. J Shoulder Elbow Surg 2007;16:388–95.

49. Koscielniak-Nielsen Z, Rasmussen H, Hesselbjerg L. Pneumothorax after an ultrasound-guided lateral sagittal infraclavicular block. Acta Anaesthesiol Scand 2008;52:1176.
50. Sites BD, Spence BC, Gallagher JD, et al. Characterizing novice behavior associated with learning ultrasound-guided peripheral regional anesthesia. Reg Anesth Pain Med 2007;32:107.
51. Fredrickson MJ, Borgeat A, Aguirre J, et al. Ultrasound-guided interscalene block should be compared with the accepted standard for the neurostimulation technique. Reg Anesth Pain Med 2009;34:18.
52. Salinas FV, Neal JM. A tale of two needle passes. Reg Anesth Pain Med 2008;33:195–8.
53. Aguirre J, Valentin Neudörfer C, Ekatodramis G, et al. Ultrasound guidance for sciatic nerve block at the popliteal fossa should be compared with the best motor response and the lowest current clinically used in neurostimulation technique. Reg Anesth Pain Med 2009;34:182–3.
54. Perlas A, Niazi A, McCartney C, et al. The sensitivity of motor response to nerve stimulation and paresthesia for nerve localization as evaluated by ultrasound. Reg Anesth Pain Med 2006;31:445–50.
55. Beach ML, Sites BD, Gallagher JD. Use of a nerve stimulator does not improve the efficacy of ultrasound-guided supraclavicular nerve blocks. J Clin Anesth 2006;18:580–4.
56. Brown DL. Atlas of regional anesthesia. 3rd edition. Philadelphia: Elsevier Saunders; 2006. p. 51.
57. Sites BD, Chan VW, Neal JM, et al. The American Society of Regional Anesthesia and Pain Medicine and the European Society of Regional Anaesthesia and Pain Therapy joint committee recommendations for education and training in ultrasound-guided regional anesthesia. Reg Anesth Pain Med 2009;34:40–6.
58. Exadaktylos AK, Buggy DJ, Moriarty DC, et al. Can anesthetic technique for primary breast cancer surgery affect recurrence or metastasis? Anesthesiology 2006;4:660–4.

Continuous Peripheral Nerve Blocks in the Hospital and at Home

Brian M. Ilfeld, MD, MS

KEYWORDS

- Continuous peripheral nerve block
- Perineural local anesthetic infusion • Postoperative analgesia
- Continuous catheter

A single-injection peripheral nerve block using long-acting local anesthetic will provide analgesia for 12 to 24 hours; however, many surgical procedures result in pain that lasts far longer. One relatively new option is a continuous peripheral nerve block (CPNB), also called "perineural local anesthetic infusion." This technique involves the percutaneous insertion of a catheter directly adjacent to the peripheral nerve(s) supplying the surgical site (as opposed to a "wound" catheter placed directly at a surgical site). Infusing local anesthetic via the perineural catheter then provides potent, site-specific analgesia. This method was first described in 1946 using a cork to stabilize a needle placed adjacent to the brachial plexus divisions to provide a "continuous" supraclavicular block.[1] Subsequently, Sarnoff and Sarnoff[2] described the use of an indwelling plastic catheter allowing repeated boluses of local anesthetic along the phrenic nerve to treat intractable hiccups. Additional sporadic techniques and applications of CPNB were reported,[3–5] but it was not until the 1990s that technological advances in needle technology, placement techniques (eg, nerve stimulators), catheter design, and infusion pump mechanics presaged a plethora of CPNB research activity.[6,7]

INDICATIONS AND SELECTION CRITERIA

Because not all patients desire, or are capable of accepting, the extra responsibility that comes with the catheter and pump system, appropriate patient selection is crucial

Funding: This work was supported by the Department of Anesthesiology, University of California San Diego, San Diego, California.

Conflict of Interest: Dr Ilfeld has received research funding from multiple companies that manufacture and/or distribute portable infusion pumps and perineural catheters. No company had any input into any aspect of this article's preparation.

Department of Anesthesiology, University of California San Diego, 200 West Arbor Drive, MC 8770, San Diego, CA 92103-8770, USA
E-mail address: bilfeld@ucsd.edu

Anesthesiology Clin 29 (2011) 193–211
doi:10.1016/j.anclin.2011.04.003
1932-2275/11/$ – see front matter © 2011 Elsevier Inc. All rights reserved.

for safe CPNB, particularly in the ambulatory environment.[8] Patients with known hepatic or renal insufficiency are often excluded in an effort to avoid local anesthetic toxicity.[9] For interscalene and cervical paravertebral infusions that may affect the phrenic nerve and ipsilateral diaphragm function,[10] particular caution is warranted in patients with heart or lung disease who may not be able to compensate for mild hypercarbia and/or hypoxia.[11]

Because there are inherent risks with any invasive procedure,[12,13] most practitioners limit the use of CPNB to patients expected to have postoperative pain lasting longer than 12 to 24 hours that is not easily managed with oral analgesics. However, CPNB has been used following *mildly* painful procedures to decrease opioid requirements and related side effects.[14,15] There are few published data on the use of various catheter locations for specific surgical procedures, although individual recommendations are available (**Table 1**).[16] In general, axillary, cervical paravertebral (CPVB), infraclavicular, or supraclavicular infusions are used for surgical procedures involving the hand, wrist, forearm, or elbow; interscalene, CPVB, and intersternocleidomastoid catheters are used for surgical procedures involving the shoulder or proximal humerus; thoracic paravertebral catheters are used for breast or other thoracic/abdominal procedures; psoas compartment catheters are used for hip surgery; fascia iliaca, femoral, and psoas compartment catheters are used for knee or thigh procedures; and popliteal/subgluteal catheters are used for surgical procedures of the leg, ankle, or foot.

EQUIPMENT AND TECHNIQUES
Techniques and Approaches

Although there are numerous catheter-placement techniques reported, from ultrasound[17,18] and fluoroscopic guidance[19] to nerve stimulation[20] and listening for a fascial "click,"[21] few studies specifically address the question of which technique is optimal for the various catheter locations. Although many proponents voice firm opinions based on their experience and/or imaging studies, few clinical data exist. Therefore, the optimal approach for catheter placement at each anatomic location remains unknown and deserves future study.

Stimulating versus Nonstimulating Catheters

One common technique involves giving a bolus of local anesthetic via an insulated needle (attached to a nerve stimulator) to provide a surgical block, followed by the introduction of a "nonstimulating" catheter.[22] However, in using this technique, it is

Table 1
Common catheter insertions for surgical procedures on various anatomic locations (recommended site underlined)

Surgical Procedure Location	Catheter Insertion Location
Shoulder or proximal humerus	Interscalene, intersternocleidomastoid, cervical paravertebral
Distal humerus, elbow, forearm, hand	Supraclavicular, infraclavicular, axillary
Breast, thoracic, or abdominal incisions	Paravertebral
Hip	Psoas compartment (posterior lumbar plexus), fascia iliaca, and femoral
Thigh and knee	Fascia iliaca and femoral
Leg, ankle, and foot	Subgluteal and popliteal sciatic

possible to provide a successful surgical block, but inaccurate catheter placement.[23] Some practitioners first insert the catheter and then administer a bolus of local anesthetic via the catheter in an effort to avoid this problem, with a reported failure rate of 1% to 8%.[24,25] Alternatively, catheters that deliver current to their tips have been developed in an attempt to improve initial placement success rates.[7] These catheters provide feedback on the positional relationship of the catheter tip to the target nerve before local anesthetic dosing.[26] There are limited data suggesting that stimulating catheters may, under some conditions, provide superior analgesia.[27] Regardless of the equipment/technique used, a "test dose" of local anesthetic with epinephrine should be administered via the catheter in an effort to identify intrathecal, epidural, or intravascular placement before infusion initiation. Ultrasound guidance is quickly gaining adherents, and may soon render the "stimulating versus nonstimulating" catheter debate moot.

Ultrasound-Guided Catheter Insertion

For ultrasound-guided procedures, the term "long axis" is used when the length of a nerve is within the ultrasound beam, compared with "short axis" when viewed in cross section.[18] A needle inserted with its length within a 2-dimensional ultrasound beam is described as "in plane," whereas a needle inserted across a 2-dimensional ultrasound beam is termed "out of plane."[18] Catheter insertion may be achieved with 3 various techniques, which are described in the following sections.

Needle out-of-plane, nerve in short-axis approach
Potential benefits of this approach include a generally familiar parallel needle-to-nerve trajectory used with traditional nerve stimulation techniques (and also vascular access); and the catheter may theoretically remain in closer proximity to the nerve, even when threaded more than a centimeter past the needle tip, because the needle is parallel to the target nerve.[28,29] However, a disadvantage of this technique is the relative inability to visualize the advancing needle tip,[28,30] which some speculate increases the likelihood of unwanted contact with nerves, vessels, peritoneum, pleura, or even meninges.[31] Practitioners often use a combination of tissue movement and "hydrolocation," in which fluid is injected and the resulting expansion infers the needle tip location (either with or without color Doppler flow).[30,32] It has been suggested that for superficial catheters (eg, interscalene and femoral), the consequent "longitudinal" orientation of needle with nerve makes precise visualization of the needle tip less critical, as the needle tip tends to remain relatively close to the nerve if the needle tip is advanced beyond the ultrasound beam. However, for deeper nerves, this technique is not as straightforward as guiding the needle tip to a target nerve, as in the in-plane technique, and may be more difficult to master (and, at times, nearly impossible).[33,34]

Needle in-plane, nerve in short-axis approach
Because this view allows for easier nerve identification, this is the most-frequently published *single*-injection peripheral nerve block orientation.[18] The needle tip location can be more easily identified relative to the target nerve when the long axis of the needle is inserted within the ultrasound plane. If the initial local anesthetic bolus is placed through the needle, its spread may be directly observed and needle tip adjustments made, when necessary. However, the perineural catheter tends to bypass the nerve during insertion, given the perpendicular orientation of the block needle and target nerve,[35] although there are certain anatomic locations that will often allow a catheter to be passed and remain perineural.[36,37] Some practitioners have advocated either passing the catheter a minimal distance past the needle tip, or advancing the catheter further initially and

then, after needle removal, retracting the catheter such that its orifice(s) lies a minimal distance (<2 cm) past the original needle tip position.[28] Some advocate using an extremely flexible perineural catheter in an attempt to keep the catheter tip in close proximity to the target nerve if the catheter is inserted more than a minimal distance.[38,39] Still others describe reorienting the needle from an in-plane to a more parallel trajectory and inserting a stimulating catheter to better monitor catheter tip location.[40]

There are multiple benefits of the needle in-plane, nerve in short-axis approach. Practitioners may learn only one technique because it may be used for both single-injection and catheter insertion procedures. In addition, it may be used for nearly all anatomic catheter locations, even for deeper target nerves.[41] There are disadvantages of this approach as well. They include new needle entry sites relative to the nerve compared with more traditional nerve-stimulation modalities that typically use a parallel needle-to-nerve insertion; challenges keeping the needle shaft in-plane[42]; difficult needle tip visualization for relatively deep nerves[33,34]; and, as noted previously, the catheter tip may bypass the target nerve given the perpendicular orientation of the needle and nerve.[35] If an extremely flexible catheter is used in an attempt to minimize this issue, it is sometimes difficult to thread past the tip of the placement needle.[38,39]

Needle in-plane and nerve in long-axis approach

Superficially, this technique appears to have the benefits of both previously described approaches, with few limitations. The nerve can be viewed along with the needle shaft/tip, and the catheter monitored as it exits the needle parallel to the target nerve. The difficulty lies in keeping 3 structures—the needle, nerve, and catheter—in the ultrasound plane.[43,44] In addition, to view the nerve in long axis, the nerve itself must be relatively straight, and there can be only one target nerve as opposed to multiple trunks or cords, as found within the brachial plexus. Evidence of this technique's difficulties may be found in the scarcity of reports.[43–45]

Limitations on the length of this article precludes a discussion of multiple additional ultrasound-related issues, such as transducer selection, the concomitant use of nerve stimulation (an important tool in a subset of patients),[46] and various methods for catheter tip localization.[47] Although many proponents voice firm opinions based on their personal experience, few clinical data exist comparing aspects of any one placement technique with another.

INFUSATES

Currently, there is insufficient information to determine if there is an optimal local anesthetic for CPNB. Although levobupivacaine and shorter-acting agents have been used, most investigators use bupivacaine or ropivacaine. Studies involving one may not be applied to another because these local anesthetics have varying durations of action.[48] One trial involving interscalene infusion found that ropivacaine 0.2% and bupivacaine 0.15% provide similar analgesia, but ropivacaine was associated with better preservation of strength in the hand and less paresthesia in the fingers,[48] although other studies comparing ropivacaine and either levobupivacaine[49] or bupivacaine[15] found no difference. Given that the equipotent local anesthetic concentrations within the peripheral nervous system remain undetermined, evaluation of comparisons is problematic. Based on preliminary evidence, it appears that the total local anesthetic dose, as opposed to concentration or delivery rate, mainly determines infusion effects,[50] although the data are somewhat conflicting.[51–54] For ropivacaine and bupivacaine, concentrations between 0.1% and 0.2% and 0.1% and 0.125% are most commonly used, respectively. Regarding additives, opioids and epinephrine have been used,[55,56] but there are currently insufficient published data to draw any conclusions regarding the safety of the former[57] or the efficacy of the latter.[58,59] And although clonidine has been often added to long-acting local anesthetic in perineural infusions,[60-65] 3 randomized, double-masked, placebo-controlled trials have failed to reveal any clinically relevant benefits.[66-68]

LOCAL ANESTHETIC DELIVERY STRATEGIES

Unfortunately, there is no single optimal local anesthetic delivery regimen.[51-53,61,63,64,69-75] In general, providing a basal infusion minimizes breakthrough pain and sleep disturbances.[64,69,70,75] Adding patient-controlled bolus doses improves analgesia, decreases opioids and related side effects, and allows for a lower basal infusion rate,[69,70] although there are exceptions.[61,75] Lowering the basal infusion rate may decrease the risk of patient falls for catheters that influence quadriceps femoris strength, such as femoral, fascia iliaca, and psoas compartment infusions (Brian Ilfeld, MD, MS, unpublished data, 2010). Unfortunately, insufficient information is available to base recommendations on the optimal basal rate, bolus volume, and lockout period, which accounts for the many variables that may effect these values (eg, catheter type, location, surgical procedure). Until recommendations based on prospectively collected data are published, practitioners may consider using the following *initial* settings with long-acting local anesthetics: basal rate of 4 to 8 mL/h (low end of range for lower extremity infusions), bolus volume of 2 to 5 mL, and lockout duration of 20 to 60 minutes. In addition, it is of great value to be able to adjust the basal infusion rate, as there is no way to predict each patient's requirements in advance, and surgical pain decreases as time progresses.[76]

AMBULATORY INFUSION

Although many issues are similar between hospital-based and outpatient CPNB, such as catheter insertion techniques, ambulatory perineural infusion poses some distinct challenges requiring some unique solutions. For example, time pressures are often more intense at high-turnover ambulatory centers, and ultrasound-guided catheter insertion not only decreases the median/mean time for placement across all subjects, but also essentially eliminates the few patients who require more than 10 minutes for catheter insertion (unlike nerve-stimulation techniques).[39,41,77,78] In addition, secondary block failure may occur following discharge, so identifying inaccurately placed perineural catheters during insertion becomes even more critical.[8,23] As noted previously, but deserving special emphasis for ambulatory infusions because not all patients desire, or are capable of accepting, the extra responsibility that comes with the catheter and pump system, appropriate patient selection is crucial for safe CPNB.[8] Patients with known hepatic or renal insufficiency are often excluded in an effort to avoid local anesthetic toxicity.[9] For interscalene and cervical paravertebral infusions that may affect the phrenic nerve and ipsilateral diaphragm function,[10] particular caution is warranted in obese individuals and patients with heart or lung disease who may not be able to compensate for mild hypercarbia and/or hypoxia.[11]

Infusion Pump Selection

In general, electronic infusion pumps provide highly accurate (90%–100% expected) and consistent (±5% baseline) basal rates over the entire infusion duration.[79-82] Elastomeric devices generally provide a higher-than-expected basal rate initially (110%–125% expected), returning to their expected rate within 2 to 12 hours, and again increasing to a higher rate before reservoir exhaustion.[8] Similarly, spring-powered pumps initially provide a higher-than-expected basal rate (115%–135% expected), which steadily decreases to a lower-than-expected rate (70%–75% expected) by reservoir exhaustion.[8] Currently, there are insufficient published data to determine the clinical situations in which the typical basal rate variation of nonelectronic pumps would be clinically relevant. As noted previously, a variable basal rate and patient-controlled bolus dose provide perineural infusion benefits, and are probably even more important in the ambulatory setting: by providing bolus doses, the basal rate may be decreased, greatly increasing the duration of infusion before reservoir exhaustion. In addition, as patients' surgical pain resolves with time, the basal rate may be decreased, also enabling the maximum infusion duration before reservoir exhaustion.[76] Reservoir volume should usually be at least 400 and 500 mL for lower-extremity and upper-extremity infusions, respectively, providing 2 to 3 days of analgesia. Electronic infusion pumps make a "click" every time they infuse (often more than twice per minute), which may prove disturbing to patients trying to sleep. Last, there are some electronic infusion pumps that have internal batteries that may not be removed. It is illegal in some locations (eg, the states of California and New York) to dispose of such pumps in the standard garbage, and special pump-delivery protocols must be set up for outpatients.

Discharge

Patients and their caretakers should be educated regarding the infusion pump and catheter system before discharge, because most patients have some degree of postoperative cognitive dysfunction. Both verbal *and written* instructions should be provided, along with contact numbers for health care providers who are available throughout the infusion duration. Along with standard postoperative outpatient instructions, topics reviewed usually include infusion pump instructions, expectations regarding surgical block resolution, breakthrough pain treatment, limb protection, bathing instructions, explicit direction to avoid driving, education that leakage at the catheter site is not dangerous (use hand towels to absorb fluid), and catheter removal plan.[8]

It is currently impossible to accurately *predict* which patients will require oral opioids. Therefore, a prescription for oral analgesics should be provided to all patients, and the importance of filling the prescription immediately after leaving the surgical center should be emphasized. A period of inadequate analgesia may result if patients wait to fill the prescription until after they have determined if oral analgesics are required. Patients discharged home must be able to ambulate. Therefore, discharge with a lower-extremity peripheral nerve block remains controversial. Although there is published evidence that discharge with an insensate extremity following a single-injection nerve block results in minimal complications,[83] there are multiple case reports of falls during lower-extremity CPNB,[84–87] and the specific incidence remains unknown. Therefore, conservative management may be optimal and some investigators have recommended that patients avoid using their surgical limb for weight bearing.[8]

Home Care

Practitioners should consider documenting each patient contact, as is standard of care for inpatients. The optimal frequency of contact with ambulatory patients is currently unknown, and probably is dependent on multiple factors, such as patient comorbidities and surgical procedure. Multiple investigators have discharged patients with instructions to call with any questions or concerns; others have suggested that patients be contacted daily by telephone; whereas still others have provided twice-daily home nursing visits in addition to telephone calls. Investigators have reported catheter removal by various techniques: some discharge patients with written instructions, others have insisted on a health care provider performing this procedure, whereas others have patients' caretakers (or occasionally the patients themselves) remove the catheters with instructions given by a provider over the telephone. Although there are no data documenting the superiority of any one technique, one survey revealed that with instructions given by phone, 98% of patients felt comfortable removing their catheter at home.[88] Of note, only 4% would have preferred to return for a health care provider to remove the catheter, and 43% responded that they would have felt comfortable with exclusively written instructions. The presence of a blue/silver catheter tip identified by the person removing the catheter confirms complete removal (depending on catheter design), and should be documented in the medical record.

POTENTIAL BENEFITS

Multiple randomized, controlled studies involving patients scheduled for moderately painful surgical procedures demonstrate the potent analgesia CPNB provides.[60–62,89–97] Improved analgesia leads to dramatic decreases in required supplemental opioids, opioid-related side effects, and sleep disturbances, while simultaneously increasing patient satisfaction.[89,90,92] In addition, one study reported a decreased time to adequate ambulation and optimization of daily activities using ambulatory CPNB compared with intravenous opioids.[98] Continuous interscalene and femoral nerve blocks following shoulder and knee arthroplasty result in an accelerated resumption of tolerated passive joint range-of-motion[91,99,100]; in some cases[60,62] leading to shorter hospitalization.[91,99] Providing ambulatory continuous femoral and psoas compartment nerve blocks decreases the time until discharge readiness following knee and hip arthroplasty, although an increased incidence of patient falls in patients receiving ropivacaine versus saline through their catheters is cause for caution before instituting early discharge.[85–87] Nonetheless, ambulatory shoulder arthroplasty and 23-hour-stay knee and hip arthroplasty have been reported using ambulatory continuous interscalene, femoral, and psoas compartment nerve blocks.[101–103] Should early discharge be allowed following joint arthroplasty, hospitalization-related costs may be decreased.[103] Although post–knee arthroplasty inflammation is decreased after a continuous femoral nerve block,[104] the continuous block has failed to produce major improvements in long-term outcomes such as decreased chronic pain and improved health-related quality of life.[105,106]

POTENTIAL RISKS/COMPLICATIONS

Two of the largest prospective investigations to date involving more than 2100 patients combined suggest that the incidence of related complications is very low—at least as low as, if not lower than, single-injection techniques.[24,107] Smaller studies involving continuous infraclavicular and popliteal blocks suggest a similar incidence of complications.[25,108]

Inaccurate Catheter Placement

The initial bolus of local anesthetic placed via the needle may produce a successful nerve block; but the catheter tip may be inaccurately placed, resulting in what has been called "secondary block failure."[22,23] The incidence of this complication is 0% to 40%,[22,23] and presumably is dependent on many factors, including the experience of the practitioner, equipment, and technique, as well as patient factors, such as body habitus.[109,110] Practitioners have first inserted the catheter and then injected the initial local anesthetic via the catheter in an effort to decrease the chances of secondary block failure.[24,26,69,70,75] If a surgical block does not develop, the catheter may be replaced. Ultrasound guidance may dramatically alter the incidence of catheter misplacement, but additional evidence must be collected to allow definitive conclusions.[39,41,77,78]

Catheter Dislodgement

Inadvertent catheter dislodgement is one of the most common complications during perineural infusion, with a reported incidence between 0% and 30%.[8] To maximize patient benefits, every effort to optimally secure the catheter must be made, especially in ambulatory patients. Measures have included the use of sterile liquid adhesive (eg, benzoin), sterile tape (eg, "Steri-Strips"), securing of the catheter-hub connection with either tape or specifically designed devices (eg, "Statlock"), subcutaneous tunneling of the catheter, and the use of 2-octyl cyanoacrylate glue (**Fig. 1**).[111] Using a combination of these maneuvers, 1-week catheter retention rates of 95% to 100% are possible.[101,112]

Vascular Puncture/Hematoma

Vascular puncture and subsequent hematoma formation is certainly a well-known complication of single-injection peripheral nerve blocks, but may be a more significant occurrence when placing a perineural catheter because the needle gauge is often larger to allow for intraluminal catheter insertion (**Fig. 2**). Using nerve stimulation and an insulated needle, the incidence of this complication is reportedly between 0% and 11%, and most likely is influenced significantly by such variables as the anatomic block location and needle/catheter design.[22,70,107,108,113,114] However, the addition of

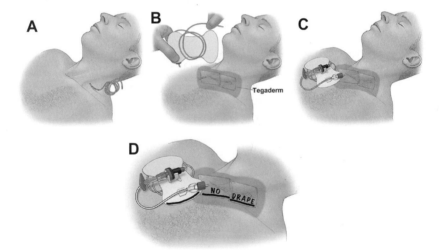

Fig. 1. Securing a perineural catheter. (*A*) An interscalene catheter placed using nerve stimulation from the anterolateral technique following needle removal. Note that any hair where an adhesive will be applied has been clipped before sterilization for the catheter insertion. (*B*) Benzoin (medical adhesive) is placed beyond the boarders of where the occlusive dressings will be placed, slightly overlapping occlusive dressings are applied, and excess catheter is wound on the back of an anchoring device. (*C*) The anchoring device is placed slightly overlapping the occlusive dressing, which will permit easy removal of all 3 adhesives on infusion discontinuation. (*D*) Surgical drapes are often inadvertently placed across clear occlusive dressings, which then remove the dressings following the surgical procedure, contaminating (or dislodging) the catheter. Outlining the dressings and communicating with the surgeon ("no drape") will help avoid this scenario.

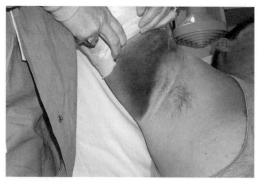

Fig. 2. A hematoma following axillary artery puncture with a 17-gauge needle during a nerve stimulation guided infraclavicular block and perineural catheter insertion. The hematoma resolved within 6 weeks, without negative sequelae.

ultrasound guidance may significantly decrease the risk of entering a vessel.[39,41,77,78] Following interscalene catheter insertion, a prolonged Horner syndrome owing to neck hematoma has been reported, but is very rare.[12] Although a hematoma may require weeks for resolution (months for a Horner syndrome), practitioners and patients should be reassured with the multiple case reports of complete neural recovery following hematoma resolution.[12,113,115,116] If vascular puncture occurs, it is still possible to successfully place a perineural catheter using nerve stimulation following a period of direct pressure, although a resulting hematoma will conduct electrical current and may decrease the ability to stimulate the target nerve with subsequent attempts.[70] Of note, clinically significant hematoma formation has been reported in patients with a psoas compartment catheter who received low molecular weight heparin (LMWH) for anticoagulation.[115,116] These occurrences have led some practitioners to manage patients with a psoas compartment catheter in much the same way as those having neuraxial block when thromboprophylaxis is ordered,[115] although others have questioned this practice.[117] The Second American Society of Regional Anesthesia consensus statement on neuraxial anesthesia and anticoagulation notes that, "conservatively, the [recommendations]… may be applied to plexus and peripheral techniques. However, this may be more restrictive than necessary," and "additional information is needed to make definitive recommendations."[118(p192)] Few substantial revisions to these recommendations were included in the more-recent Third Consensus Statement.[119]

Delayed Local Anesthetic Toxicity

Patients have reported early symptoms of local anesthetic toxicity during CPNB (eg, perioral numbness) that resolved with infusion termination.[120,121] Although practitioners should remain alert to the possibility of this complication, it remains an extraordinarily rare event. The maximum safe doses for the long-acting local anesthetics as well as the incidence of systemic toxicity are unknown; however, infusing 40 mg or less of ropivacaine each hour has resulted in a remarkably rare incidence of toxicity events, even over the course of multiple weeks.[122] Of note, providing patients with the ability to self-administer bolus doses decreases local anesthetic consumption.[61,63,64,69–71,73–76,123] Related to this, investigators often exclude patients from an ambulatory or long-duration CPNB with known hepatic or renal insufficiency in an effort to avoid local anesthetic toxicity.[9,89,90,92]

Nerve Injury

Nerve injury is a recognized complication following placement of both single-injection and CPNB, presumably related to needle trauma and/or subsequent local anesthetic/adjuvant neurotoxicity.[124] Current evidence suggests that the incidence of neural injury from a perineural catheter and ropivacaine (0.2%) infusion is no higher than following single-injection regional blocks.[24,25,113,121] There are 2 case reports of interscalene perineural catheters possibly resulting in brachial plexus irritation.[13] In both of these cases, repeated boluses of 0.25% bupivacaine had been injected over a period of days, and patient discomfort ceased upon removal of the catheters.[13] There is also evidence that in diabetes, the risk of local anesthetic-induced nerve injury is increased.[125]

Infection

Clinically relevant catheter-related infection remains an uncommon occurrence, even though catheter site bacterial colonization is relatively common.[107,113,126,127] In more than 2700 patients combined, infection rates varied from 0% to 3%, with one psoas compartment abscess forming following femoral CPNB in prospective investigations of interscalene,[24,113] posterior popliteal,[25] and multiple-site[107] catheters. In these few cases, all infections completely resolved within 10 days, and there has never been a reported case of a permanent deficit caused by a catheter infection.[107,128] Although there are cases of prolonged infusions lasting many weeks,[122] limiting catheter use to 3 to 4 days may further decrease the incidence of this complication,[107] and practitioners should balance the need for analgesia with the risk of infection.[127] Although data specific for perineural catheters are lacking, current guidelines recommend treating catheter insertion with the same sterile precautions as central lines, including use of a sterilization solution (eg, chlorhexidine) at the insertion site, sterile gloves, and drape, as well as a hat and mask. Although some practitioners wear a sterile gown during catheter insertion, this addition is currently somewhat controversial.

Perineuraxis Injection

It is possible to cannulate the epidural[129–131] or intrathecal[132] spaces when placing a catheter near the neuraxis, as with the psoas compartment and interscalene locations. Potentially catastrophic is the injection of local anesthetic, which may result in unconsciousness and extreme hypotension requiring aggressive resuscitation. As with intravascular catheter placement, it is possible to accurately inject the initial bolus of local anesthetic via the needle, followed by cannulation of the epidural,[129] intrathecal,[132] and even intrapleural spaces with the catheter.[133] Of note, when working close to the neuraxis, it is possible to get epidural local anesthetic spread even with an accurately placed perineural catheter, resulting in a sympathectomy and possible hypotension. Whether ultrasound guidance will result in a decreased incidence of such complications is currently unknown, given the relatively recent advent of ultrasound-guided perineural catheter insertion.

Catheter Migration

Spontaneous migration into adjacent anatomic structures following a documented correct placement has been described in only one patient.[107] Possible theoretical complications from such an incident include intravascular or interpleural migration resulting in local anesthetic toxicity, and epidural/intrathecal migration when using an interscalene, intersternocleidomastoid, paravertebral, or psoas compartment catheter. Of note, it is possible to accidentally position the catheter tip in the epidural space (and presumably other structures) following partial catheter withdrawl.[129]

Pulmonary Complications

For infusions that may affect the phrenic nerve and ipsilateral diaphragm function (eg, interscalene or cervical paravertebral catheters), caution is warranted, as interscalene CPNBs have been shown to cause frequent ipsilateral diaphragm paralysis.[11] Although the effect on overall pulmonary function may be minimal for relatively healthy patients,[10] a case of clinically relevant lower lobe collapse in a patient with an interscalene infusion at home and 2 cases of acute respiratory failure have occurred.[107,134]

Catheter Knotting and Retention

Several case reports of catheter retention have been published, although the overall incidence of this complication is unknown.[70,135–137] The most common etiology is knot formation below the skin or fascia, and has been reported in fascia iliaca,[135] femoral,[136] and psoas compartment catheters.[137] Two of these cases required surgical exploration for catheter removal[136,137]; however, removal of a knotted fascia iliaca catheter was achieved without surgical intervention with simple hip flexion.[135] In all of these cases, the catheter had been advanced more than 5 cm past the needle tip. Advancing the catheter more than 3 to 5 cm is often attempted in an effort to decrease the risk of dislodgement, or to "thread" the catheter tip toward the lumbar plexus when using the femoral or fascia iliaca insertion points.[138] However, retention rates of 95% to 100% have been reported using a maximum distance of 5 cm[66,67,69,70,75,89,90,92], and in the absence of using a catheter-over-wire Seldinger technique,[61–63,139,140] the catheter tip rarely reaches the lumbar plexus following a femoral insertion.[138] The available data suggest that insertion greater than 5 cm is unnecessary and may increase the knotting risk, although there is no consensus regarding the optimal distance of catheter insertion.[135]

Catheter Shearing

It is possible to "shear off" a segment of catheter if, following insertion past the needle tip, the catheter itself is withdrawn back into the needle. Therefore, this maneuver should be attempted only when using needle/catheter combinations that have been specifically designed for catheter withdrawal. And when using specifically designed needle/catheter combinations, such as with some stimulating catheters, catheter withdrawal should cease with any resistance, and the needle itself retracted until the catheter resistance resolves.[67,69,70,75,141] In one reported case, a 6-cm femoral catheter fragment was sheared off and remained in situ for 1 week, causing persistent pain of the ipsilateral groin, thigh, and knee.[142] Despite an embedded radiopaque strip, the catheter fragment could not be visualized with plain radiographs. However, a computerized tomographic scan did localize the fragment and the femoral nerve neuralgia resolved in the week following surgical extraction of the fragment.[142] In an additional case, an axillary catheter fragment was diagnosed with ultrasonography and surgically extracted.[121] In all of the case reports of retained catheters/fragments, no patient experienced persistent symptoms following removal.[70,121,141,142]

REFERENCES

1. Ansbro FP. A method of continuous brachial plexus block. Am J Surg 1946;71: 716–22.

2. Sarnoff SJ, Sarnoff LC. Prolonged peripheral nerve block by means of indwelling plastic catheter. Treatment of hiccup. Anesthesiology 1951;12:270–5.
3. Cheeley LN. Treatment of peripheral embolism by continuous sciatic nerve block. Curr Res Anesth Analg 1952;31:211–2.
4. Manriquez RG, Pallares V. Continuous brachial plexus block for prolonged sympathectomy and control of pain. Anesth Analg 1978;57:128–30.
5. DeKrey JA, Schroeder CF, Buechel DR. Continuous brachial plexus block. Anesthesiology 1969;30:332.
6. Steele SM, Klein SM, D'Ercole FJ, et al. A new continuous catheter delivery system. Anesth Analg 1998;87:228.
7. Boezaart AP, de Beer JF, du TC, et al. A new technique of continuous interscalene nerve block. Can J Anaesth 1999;46:275–81.
8. Ilfeld BM, Enneking FK. Continuous peripheral nerve blocks at home: a review. Anesth Analg 2005;100:1822–33.
9. Denson DD, Raj PP, Saldahna F, et al. Continuous perineural infusion of bupivacaine for prolonged analgesia: pharmacokinetic considerations. Int J Clin Pharmacol Ther Toxicol 1983;21:591–7.
10. Borgeat A, Perschak H, Bird P, et al. Patient-controlled interscalene analgesia with ropivacaine 0.2% versus patient-controlled intravenous analgesia after major shoulder surgery: effects on diaphragmatic and respiratory function. Anesthesiology 2000;92:102–8.
11. Pere P. The effect of continuous interscalene brachial plexus block with 0.125% bupivacaine plus fentanyl on diaphragmatic motility and ventilatory function. Reg Anesth 1993;18:93–7.
12. Ekatodramis G, Macaire P, Borgeat A. Prolonged Horner syndrome due to neck hematoma after continuous interscalene block. Anesthesiology 2001;95:801–3.
13. Ribeiro FC, Georgousis H, Bertram R, et al. Plexus irritation caused by interscalene brachial plexus catheter for shoulder surgery. Anesth Analg 1996;82:870–2.
14. Rawal N, Axelsson K, Hylander J, et al. Postoperative patient-controlled local anesthetic administration at home. Anesth Analg 1998;86:86–9.
15. Rawal N, Allvin R, Axelsson K, et al. Patient-controlled regional analgesia (PCRA) at home: controlled comparison between bupivacaine and ropivacaine brachial plexus analgesia. Anesthesiology 2002;96:1290–6.
16. Boezaart AP. Perineural infusion of local anesthetics. Anesthesiology 2006;104:872–80.
17. Guzeldemir ME, Ustunsoz B. Ultrasonographic guidance in placing a catheter for continuous axillary brachial plexus block. Anesth Analg 1995;81:882–3.
18. Gray AT. Ultrasound-guided regional anesthesia: current state of the art. Anesthesiology 2006;104:368–73.
19. Pham-Dang C, Meunier JF, Poirier P, et al. A new axillary approach for continuous brachial plexus block. A clinical and anatomic study. Anesth Analg 1995;81:686–93.
20. Grant SA, Nielsen KC, Greengrass RA, et al. Continuous peripheral nerve block for ambulatory surgery. Reg Anesth Pain Med 2001;26:209–14.
21. Selander D. Catheter technique in axillary plexus block. Presentation of a new method. Acta Anaesthesiol Scand 1977;21:324–9.
22. Klein SM, Grant SA, Greengrass RA, et al. Interscalene brachial plexus block with a continuous catheter insertion system and a disposable infusion pump. Anesth Analg 2000;91:1473–8.
23. Salinas FV. Location, location, location: continuous peripheral nerve blocks and stimulating catheters. Reg Anesth Pain Med 2003;28:79–82.

24. Borgeat A, Dullenkopf A, Ekatodramis G, et al. Evaluation of the lateral modified approach for continuous interscalene block after shoulder surgery. Anesthesiology 2003;99:436–42.
25. Borgeat A, Blumenthal S, Karovic D, et al. Clinical evaluation of a modified posterior anatomical approach to performing the popliteal block. Reg Anesth Pain Med 2004;29:290–6.
26. Pham-Dang C, Kick O, Collet T, et al. Continuous peripheral nerve blocks with stimulating catheters. Reg Anesth Pain Med 2003;28:83–8.
27. Morin AM, Kranke P, Wulf H, et al. The effect of stimulating versus nonstimulating catheter techniques for continuous regional anesthesia: a semiquantitative systematic review. Reg Anesth Pain Med 2010;35:194–9.
28. Fredrickson MJ, Ball CM, Dalgleish AJ, et al. A prospective randomized comparison of ultrasound and neurostimulation as needle end points for interscalene catheter placement. Anesth Analg 2009;108:1695–700.
29. Fredrickson MJ, Danesh-Clough TK. Ambulatory continuous femoral analgesia for major knee surgery: a randomised study of ultrasound-guided femoral catheter placement. Anaesth Intensive Care 2009;37:758–66.
30. Fredrickson M. "Oblique" needle-probe alignment to facilitate ultrasound-guided femoral catheter placement. Reg Anesth Pain Med 2008;33:383–4.
31. Luyet C, Eichenberger U, Greif R, et al. Ultrasound-guided paravertebral puncture and placement of catheters in human cadavers: an imaging study. Br J Anaesth 2009;102:534–9.
32. Bloc S, Ecoffey C, Dhonneur G. Controlling needle tip progression during ultrasound-guided regional anesthesia using the hydrolocalization technique. Reg Anesth Pain Med 2008;33:382–3.
33. Chin KJ, Perlas A, Chan VW, et al. Needle visualization in ultrasound-guided regional anesthesia: challenges and solutions. Reg Anesth Pain Med 2008;33: 532–44.
34. Sites BD, Brull R, Chan VW, et al. Artifacts and pitfall errors associated with ultrasound-guided regional anesthesia. Part II: a pictorial approach to understanding and avoidance. Reg Anesth Pain Med 2007;32:419–33.
35. Dhir S, Ganapathy S. Comparative evaluation of ultrasound-guided continuous infraclavicular brachial plexus block with stimulating catheter and traditional technique: a prospective-randomized trial. Acta Anaesthesiol Scand 2008;52: 1158–66.
36. Mariano ER, Loland VJ, Ilfeld BM. Interscalene perineural catheter placement using an ultrasound-guided posterior approach. Reg Anesth Pain Med 2009;34:60–3.
37. van Geffen GJ, Gielen M. Ultrasound-guided subgluteal sciatic nerve blocks with stimulating catheters in children: a descriptive study. Anesth Analg 2006; 103:328–33.
38. Sandhu NS, Capan LM. Ultrasound-guided infraclavicular brachial plexus block. Br J Anaesth 2002;89:254–9.
39. Mariano ER, Cheng GS, Choy LP, et al. Electrical stimulation versus ultrasound guidance for popliteal-sciatic perineural catheter insertion: a randomized, controlled trial. Reg Anesth Pain Med 2009;34:480–5.
40. Niazi AU, Prasad A, Ramlogan R, et al. Methods to ease placement of stimulating catheters during in-plane ultrasound-guided femoral nerve block. Reg Anesth Pain Med 2009;34:380–1.
41. Mariano ER, Loland VJ, Bellars RH, et al. Ultrasound guidance versus electrical stimulation for infraclavicular brachial plexus perineural catheter insertion. J Ultrasound Med 2009;28:1211–8.

42. Sites BD, Spence BC, Gallagher JD, et al. Characterizing novice behavior associated with learning ultrasound-guided peripheral regional anesthesia. Reg Anesth Pain Med 2007;32:107–15.

43. Koscielniak-Nielsen ZJ, Rasmussen H, Hesselbjerg L. Long-axis ultrasound imaging of the nerves and advancement of perineural catheters under direct vision: a preliminary report of four cases. Reg Anesth Pain Med 2008;33: 477–82.

44. Wang AZ, Gu L, Zhou QH, et al. Ultrasound-guided continuous femoral nerve block for analgesia after total knee arthroplasty: catheter perpendicular to the nerve versus catheter parallel to the nerve. Reg Anesth Pain Med 2010;35: 127–31.

45. Tsui BC, Ozelsel TJ. Ultrasound-guided anterior sciatic nerve block using a longitudinal approach: "expanding the view." Reg Anesth Pain Med 2008; 33:275–6.

46. Fredrickson MJ. The sensitivity of motor response to needle nerve stimulation during ultrasound guided interscalene catheter placement. Reg Anesth Pain Med 2008;33:291–6.

47. Swenson JD, Davis JJ, DeCou JA. A novel approach for assessing catheter position after ultrasound-guided placement of continuous interscalene block. Anesth Analg 2008;106:1015–6.

48. Borgeat A, Kalberer F, Jacob H, et al. Patient-controlled interscalene analgesia with ropivacaine 0.2% versus bupivacaine 0.15% after major open shoulder surgery: the effects on hand motor function. Anesth Analg 2001;92:218–23.

49. Casati A, Borghi B, Fanelli G, et al. Interscalene brachial plexus anesthesia and analgesia for open shoulder surgery: a randomized, double-blinded comparison between levobupivacaine and ropivacaine. Anesth Analg 2003;96:253–9.

50. Ilfeld BM, Moeller LK, Mariano ER, et al. Continuous peripheral nerve blocks: is local anesthetic dose the only factor, or do concentration and volume influence infusion effects as well? Anesthesiology 2010;112:347–54.

51. Ilfeld BM, Loland VJ, Gerancher JC, et al. The effects of varying local anesthetic concentration and volume on continuous popliteal sciatic nerve blocks: a dual-center, randomized, controlled study. Anesth Analg 2008;107:701–7.

52. Ilfeld BM, Le LT, Ramjohn J, et al. The effects of local anesthetic concentration and dose on continuous infraclavicular nerve blocks: a multicenter, randomized, observer-masked, controlled study. Anesth Analg 2009;108:345–50.

53. Le LT, Loland VJ, Mariano ER, et al. Effects of local anesthetic concentration and dose on continuous interscalene nerve blocks: a dual-center, randomized, observer-masked, controlled study. Reg Anesth Pain Med 2008;33:518–25.

54. Brodner G, Buerkle H, Van Aken H, et al. Postoperative analgesia after knee surgery: a comparison of three different concentrations of ropivacaine for continuous femoral nerve blockade. Anesth Analg 2007;105:256–62.

55. Wajima Z, Shitara T, Nakajima Y, et al. Comparison of continuous brachial plexus infusion of butorphanol, mepivacaine and mepivacaine-butorphanol mixtures for postoperative analgesia. Br J Anaesth 1995;75:548–51.

56. Wajima Z, Nakajima Y, Kim C, et al. IV compared with brachial plexus infusion of butorphanol for postoperative analgesia. Br J Anaesth 1995;74:392–5.

57. Partridge BL. The effects of local anesthetics and epinephrine on rat sciatic nerve blood flow. Anesthesiology 1991;75:243–50.

58. Picard PR, Tramer MR, McQuay HJ, et al. Analgesic efficacy of peripheral opioids (all except intra-articular): a qualitative systematic review of randomised controlled trials. Pain 1997;72:309–18.

59. Murphy DB, McCartney CJ, Chan VW. Novel analgesic adjuncts for brachial plexus block: a systematic review. Anesth Analg 2000;90:1122–8.
60. Capdevila X, Barthelet Y, Biboulet P, et al. Effects of perioperative analgesic technique on the surgical outcome and duration of rehabilitation after major knee surgery. Anesthesiology 1999;91:8–15.
61. Singelyn FJ, Gouverneur JM. Extended "three-in-one" block after total knee arthroplasty: continuous versus patient-controlled techniques. Anesth Analg 2000;91:176–80.
62. Singelyn FJ, Deyaert M, Joris D, et al. Effects of intravenous patient-controlled analgesia with morphine, continuous epidural analgesia, and continuous three-in-one block on postoperative pain and knee rehabilitation after unilateral total knee arthroplasty. Anesth Analg 1998;87:88–92.
63. Singelyn FJ, Vanderelst PE, Gouverneur JM. Extended femoral nerve sheath block after total hip arthroplasty: continuous versus patient-controlled techniques. Anesth Analg 2001;92:455–9.
64. Singelyn FJ, Seguy S, Gouverneur JM. Interscalene brachial plexus analgesia after open shoulder surgery: continuous versus patient-controlled infusion. Anesth Analg 1999;89:1216–20.
65. Singelyn FJ, Aye F, Gouverneur JM. Continuous popliteal sciatic nerve block: an original technique to provide postoperative analgesia after foot surgery. Anesth Analg 1997;84:383–6.
66. Ilfeld BM, Morey TE, Enneking FK. Continuous infraclavicular perineural infusion with clonidine and ropivacaine compared with ropivacaine alone: a randomized, double-blinded, controlled study. Anesth Analg 2003;97:706–12.
67. Ilfeld BM, Morey TE, Thannikary LJ, et al. Clonidine added to a continuous interscalene ropivacaine perineural infusion to improve postoperative analgesia: a randomized, double-blind, controlled study. Anesth Analg 2005;100:1172–8.
68. Casati A, Vinciguerra F, Cappelleri G, et al. Adding clonidine to the induction bolus and postoperative infusion during continuous femoral nerve block delays recovery of motor function after total knee arthroplasty. Anesth Analg 2005;100:866–72.
69. Ilfeld BM, Morey TE, Wright TW, et al. Interscalene perineural ropivacaine infusion: a comparison of two dosing regimens for postoperative analgesia. Reg Anesth Pain Med 2004;29:9–16.
70. Ilfeld BM, Morey TE, Enneking FK. Infraclavicular perineural local anesthetic infusion: a comparison of three dosing regimens for postoperative analgesia. Anesthesiology 2004;100:395–402.
71. Iskandar H, Rakotondriamihary S, Dixmerias F, et al. Analgesia using continuous axillary block after surgery of severe hand injuries: self-administration versus continuous injection. Ann Fr Anesth Reanim 1998;17:1099–103 [in French].
72. Mezzatesta JP, Scott DA, Schweitzer SA, et al. Continuous axillary brachial plexus block for postoperative pain relief. Intermittent bolus versus continuous infusion. Reg Anesth 1997;22:357–62.
73. Eledjam JJ, Cuvillon P, Capdevila X, et al. Postoperative analgesia by femoral nerve block with ropivacaine 0.2% after major knee surgery: continuous versus patient-controlled techniques. Reg Anesth Pain Med 2002;27:604–11.
74. di Benedetto P, Casati A, Bertini L. Continuous subgluteus sciatic nerve block after orthopedic foot and ankle surgery: comparison of two infusion techniques. Reg Anesth Pain Med 2002;27:168–72.
75. Ilfeld BM, Thannikary LJ, Morey TE, et al. Popliteal sciatic perineural local anesthetic infusion: a comparison of three dosing regimens for postoperative analgesia. Anesthesiology 2004;101:970–7.

76. Ilfeld BM, Enneking FK. A portable mechanical pump providing over four days of patient-controlled analgesia by perineural infusion at home. Reg Anesth Pain Med 2002;27:100–4.

77. Mariano ER, Loland VJ, Sandhu NS, et al. Ultrasound guidance versus electrical stimulation for femoral perineural catheter insertion. J Ultrasound Med 2009;28: 1453–60.

78. Mariano ER, Loland VJ, Sandhu NS, et al. A trainee-based randomized comparison of stimulating interscalene perineural catheters with a new technique using ultrasound guidance alone. J Ultrasound Med 2010;29:329–36.

79. Ilfeld BM, Morey TE, Enneking FK. The delivery rate accuracy of portable infusion pumps used for continuous regional analgesia. Anesth Analg 2002;95: 1331–6.

80. Ilfeld BM, Morey TE, Enneking FK. Delivery rate accuracy of portable, bolus-capable infusion pumps used for patient-controlled continuous regional analgesia. Reg Anesth Pain Med 2003;28:17–23.

81. Ilfeld BM, Morey TE, Enneking FK. Portable infusion pumps used for continuous regional analgesia: delivery rate accuracy and consistency. Reg Anesth Pain Med 2003;28:424–32.

82. Ilfeld BM, Morey TE, Enneking FK. New portable infusion pumps: real advantages or just more of the same in a different package? Reg Anesth Pain Med 2004;29:371–6.

83. Klein SM, Nielsen KC, Greengrass RA, et al. Ambulatory discharge after long-acting peripheral nerve blockade: 2382 blocks with ropivacaine. Anesth Analg 2002;94:65–70.

84. Williams BA, Kentor ML, Bottegal MT. The incidence of falls at home in patients with perineural femoral catheters: a retrospective summary of a randomized clinical trial. Anesth Analg 2007;104:1002.

85. Ilfeld BM, Le LT, Meyer RS, et al. Ambulatory continuous femoral nerve blocks decrease time to discharge readiness after tricompartment total knee arthroplasty: a randomized, triple-masked, placebo-controlled study. Anesthesiology 2008;108:703–13.

86. Ilfeld BM, Mariano ER, Girard PJ, et al. A multicenter, randomized, triple-masked, placebo-controlled trial of the effect of ambulatory continuous femoral nerve blocks on discharge-readiness following total knee arthroplasty in patients on general orthopaedic wards. Pain 2010;150:477–84.

87. Ilfeld BM, Ball ST, Gearen PF, et al. Ambulatory continuous posterior lumbar plexus nerve blocks after hip arthroplasty: a dual-center, randomized, triple-masked, placebo-controlled trial. Anesthesiology 2008;109:491–501.

88. Ilfeld BM, Esener DE, Morey TE, et al. Ambulatory perineural infusion: the patients' perspective. Reg Anesth Pain Med 2003;28:418–23.

89. Ilfeld BM, Morey TE, Enneking FK. Continuous infraclavicular brachial plexus block for postoperative pain control at home: a randomized, double-blinded, placebo-controlled study. Anesthesiology 2002;96:1297–304.

90. Ilfeld BM, Morey TE, Wright TW, et al. Continuous interscalene brachial plexus block for postoperative pain control at home: a randomized, double-blinded, placebo-controlled study. Anesth Analg 2003;96:1089–95.

91. Ilfeld BM, Vandenborne K, Duncan PW, et al. Ambulatory continuous interscalene nerve blocks decrease the time to discharge readiness after total shoulder arthroplasty: a randomized, triple-masked, placebo-controlled study. Anesthesiology 2006;105:999–1007.

92. Ilfeld BM, Morey TE, Wang RD, et al. Continuous popliteal sciatic nerve block for postoperative pain control at home: a randomized, double-blinded, placebo-controlled study. Anesthesiology 2002;97:959–65.

93. White PF, Issioui T, Skrivanek GD, et al. The use of a continuous popliteal sciatic nerve block after surgery involving the foot and ankle: does it improve the quality of recovery? Anesth Analg 2003;97:1303–9.

94. Ganapathy S, Wasserman RA, Watson JT, et al. Modified continuous femoral three-in-one block for postoperative pain after total knee arthroplasty. Anesth Analg 1999;89:1197–202.

95. Hirst GC, Lang SA, Dust WN, et al. Femoral nerve block. Single injection versus continuous infusion for total knee arthroplasty. Reg Anesth 1996;21:292–7.

96. Watson MW, Mitra D, McLintock T, et al. Continuous versus single-injection lumbar plexus blocks: comparison of the effects on morphine use and early recovery after total knee arthroplasty. Reg Anesth Pain Med 2005;30:541–7.

97. Borgeat A, Schappi B, Biasca N, et al. Patient-controlled analgesia after major shoulder surgery: patient-controlled interscalene analgesia versus patient-controlled analgesia. Anesthesiology 1997;87:1343–7.

98. Capdevila X, Dadure C, Bringuier S, et al. Effect of patient-controlled perineural analgesia on rehabilitation and pain after ambulatory orthopedic surgery: a multicenter randomized trial. Anesthesiology 2006;105:566–73.

99. Ilfeld BM, Wright TW, Enneking FK, et al. Joint range of motion after total shoulder arthroplasty with and without a continuous interscalene nerve block: a retrospective, case-control study. Reg Anesth Pain Med 2005;30:429–33.

100. Salinas FV, Liu SS, Mulroy MF. The effect of single-injection femoral nerve block versus continuous femoral nerve block after total knee arthroplasty on hospital length of stay and long-term functional recovery within an established clinical pathway. Anesth Analg 2006;102:1234–9.

101. Ilfeld BM, Wright TW, Enneking FK, et al. Total shoulder arthroplasty as an outpatient procedure using ambulatory perineural local anesthetic infusion: a pilot feasibility study. Anesth Analg 2005;101:1319–22.

102. Ilfeld BM, Gearen PF, Enneking FK, et al. Total hip arthroplasty as an overnight-stay procedure using an ambulatory continuous psoas compartment nerve block: a prospective feasibility study. Reg Anesth Pain Med 2006;31:113–8.

103. Ilfeld BM, Mariano ER, Williams BA, et al. Hospitalization costs of total knee arthroplasty with a continuous femoral nerve block provided only in the hospital versus on an ambulatory basis: a retrospective, case-control, cost-minimization analysis. Reg Anesth Pain Med 2007;32:46–54.

104. Martin F, Martinez V, Mazoit JX, et al. Antiinflammatory effect of peripheral nerve blocks after knee surgery: clinical and biologic evaluation. Anesthesiology 2008;109:484–90.

105. Ilfeld BM, Meyer RS, Le LT, et al. Health-related quality of life after tricompartment knee arthroplasty with and without an extended-duration continuous femoral nerve block: a prospective, 1-year follow-up of a randomized, triple-masked, placebo-controlled study. Anesth Analg 2009;108:1320–5.

106. Bost JE, Williams BA, Bottegal MT, et al. The 8-item Short-Form Health Survey and the physical comfort composite score of the quality of recovery 40-item scale provide the most responsive assessments of pain, physical function, and mental function during the first 4 days after ambulatory knee surgery with regional anesthesia. Anesth Analg 2007;105:1693–700.

107. Capdevila X, Pirat P, Bringuier S, et al. Continuous peripheral nerve blocks in hospital wards after orthopedic surgery: a multicenter prospective analysis of

the quality of postoperative analgesia and complications in 1,416 patients. Anesthesiology 2005;103:1035–45.

108. Borgeat A, Ekatodramis G, Dumont C. An evaluation of the infraclavicular block via a modified approach of the Raj technique. Anesth Analg 2001;93:436–41.

109. Nielsen KC, Guller U, Steele SM, et al. Influence of obesity on surgical regional anesthesia in the ambulatory setting: an analysis of 9,038 blocks. Anesthesiology 2005;102:181–7.

110. Coleman MM, Chan VW. Continuous interscalene brachial plexus block. Can J Anaesth 1999;46:209–14.

111. Klein SM, Nielsen KC, Buckenmaier CC III, et al. 2-octyl cyanoacrylate glue for the fixation of continuous peripheral nerve catheters. Anesthesiology 2003;98:590–1.

112. Ang ET, Lassale B, Goldfarb G. Continuous axillary brachial plexus block–a clinical and anatomical study. Anesth Analg 1984;63:680–4.

113. Borgeat A, Ekatodramis G, Kalberer F, et al. Acute and nonacute complications associated with interscalene block and shoulder surgery: a prospective study. Anesthesiology 2001;95:875–80.

114. Boezaart AP, de Beer JF, Nell ML. Early experience with continuous cervical paravertebral block using a stimulating catheter. Reg Anesth Pain Med 2003;28:406–13.

115. Weller RS, Gerancher JC, Crews JC, et al. Extensive retroperitoneal hematoma without neurologic deficit in two patients who underwent lumbar plexus block and were later anticoagulated. Anesthesiology 2003;98:581–5.

116. Klein SM, D'Ercole F, Greengrass RA, et al. Enoxaparin associated with psoas hematoma and lumbar plexopathy after lumbar plexus block. Anesthesiology 1997;87:1576–9.

117. Chelly JE, Greger JR, Casati A, et al. What has happened to evidence-based medicine? Anesthesiology 2003;99:1028–9.

118. Horlocker TT, Wedel DJ, Benzon H, et al. Regional anesthesia in the anticoagulated patient: defining the risks (the second ASRA Consensus Conference on Neuraxial Anesthesia and Anticoagulation). Reg Anesth Pain Med 2003;28:172–97.

119. Horlocker TT, Wedel DJ, Rowlingson JC, et al. Regional anesthesia in the patient receiving antithrombotic or thrombolytic therapy: American Society of Regional Anesthesia and Pain Medicine Evidence-Based Guidelines (Third Edition). Reg Anesth Pain Med 2010;35:64–101.

120. Tuominen M, Pitkanen M, Rosenberg PH. Postoperative pain relief and bupivacaine plasma levels during continuous interscalene brachial plexus block. Acta Anaesthesiol Scand 1987;31:276–8.

121. Bergman BD, Hebl JR, Kent J, et al. Neurologic complications of 405 consecutive continuous axillary catheters. Anesth Analg 2003;96:247–52.

122. Bleckner LL, Bina S, Kwon KH, et al. Serum ropivacaine concentrations and systemic local anesthetic toxicity in trauma patients receiving long-term continuous peripheral nerve block catheters. Anesth Analg 2010;110:630–4.

123. Chelly JE, Greger J, Gebhard R. Ambulatory continuous perineural infusion: are we ready? [letter; comment]. Anesthesiology 2000;93:581–2.

124. Al Nasser B, Palacios JL. Femoral nerve injury complicating continuous psoas compartment block. Reg Anesth Pain Med 2004;29:361–3.

125. Horlocker TT, O'Driscoll SW, Dinapoli RP. Recurring brachial plexus neuropathy in a diabetic patient after shoulder surgery and continuous interscalene block. Anesth Analg 2000;91:688–90.

126. Cuvillon P, Ripart J, Lalourcey L, et al. The continuous femoral nerve block catheter for postoperative analgesia: bacterial colonization, infectious rate and adverse effects. Anesth Analg 2001;93:1045–9.
127. Gaumann DM, Lennon RL, Wedel DJ. Continuous axillary block for postoperative pain management. Reg Anesth Pain Med 1988;13:77–82.
128. Adam F, Jaziri S, Chauvin M. Psoas abscess complicating femoral nerve block catheter. Anesthesiology 2003;99:230–1.
129. Cook LB. Unsuspected extradural catheterization in an interscalene block. Br J Anaesth 1991;67:473–5.
130. Mahoudeau G, Gaertner E, Launoy A, et al. Interscalenic block: accidental catheterization of the epidural space. Ann Fr Anesth Reanim 1995;14:438–41 [in French].
131. De Biasi P, Lupescu R, Burgun G, et al. Continuous lumbar plexus block: use of radiography to determine catheter tip location. Reg Anesth Pain Med 2003;28:135–9.
132. Litz RJ, Vicent O, Wiessner D, et al. Misplacement of a psoas compartment catheter in the subarachnoid space. Reg Anesth Pain Med 2004;29:60–4.
133. Souron V, Reiland Y, De Traverse A, et al. Interpleural migration of an interscalene catheter. Anesth Analg 2003;97:1200–1.
134. Sardesai AM, Chakrabarti AJ, Denny NM. Lower lobe collapse during continuous interscalene brachial plexus local anesthesia at home. Reg Anesth Pain Med 2004;29:65–8.
135. Offerdahl MR, Lennon RL, Horlocker TT. Successful removal of a knotted fascia iliaca catheter: principles of patient positioning for peripheral nerve catheter extraction. Anesth Analg 2004;99:1550–2.
136. Motamed C, Bouaziz H, Mercier FJ, et al. Knotting of a femoral catheter. Reg Anesth 1997;22:486–7.
137. MacLeod DB, Grant SA, Martin G, et al. Identification of coracoid process for infraclavicular blocks. Reg Anesth Pain Med 2003;28:485.
138. Capdevila X, Biboulet P, Morau D, et al. Continuous three-in-one block for postoperative pain after lower limb orthopedic surgery: where do the catheters go? Anesth Analg 2002;94:1001–6.
139. Singelyn FJ, Gouverneur JM. Postoperative analgesia after total hip arthroplasty: i.v. PCA with morphine, patient-controlled epidural analgesia, or continuous "3-in-1" block? A prospective evaluation by our acute pain service in more than 1,300 patients. J Clin Anesth 1999;11:550–4.
140. Singelyn FJ, Ferrant T, Malisse MF, et al. Effects of intravenous patient-controlled analgesia with morphine, continuous epidural analgesia, and continuous femoral nerve sheath block on rehabilitation after unilateral total-hip arthroplasty. Reg Anesth Pain Med 2005;30:452–7.
141. Chin KJ, Chee V. Perforation of a Pajunk stimulating catheter after traction-induced damage. Reg Anesth Pain Med 2006;31:389–90.
142. Lee BH, Goucke CR. Shearing of a peripheral nerve catheter. Anesth Analg 2000;95:760–1.

Economics and Practice Management Issues Associated With Acute Pain Management

Dennis P. Phillips, DO[a],*, Tara L. Knizner, MD[a],
Brian A. Williams, MD, MBA[b]

KEYWORDS

- Regional anesthesia • Economics of anesthesia
- PACU bypass • Acute postoperative pain

ECONOMICS AND PRACTICE MANAGEMENT ISSUES ASSOCIATED WITH ACUTE PAIN MANAGEMENT

The current global economic climate makes the wisdom of incorporating fiscal factors into the delivery of health care important. This review summarizes research outcomes related to the efficient use of perioperative pain management services. The majority of the citations in this text address ambulatory orthopedic surgical patient populations because most economic research to date has been in this area. Applying this research to broader patient populations, and to different facilities, becomes challenging. It is challenging because the economic outcomes of daily practice commonly reflect what is learned through experience rather than through the artificial economics of prospective, randomized controlled trial (RCT). Accordingly, Berwick (1996) states,

> Our work in medicine should be grounded in sound evidence, and proper designs and statistics are basic to this quest. But, buried in our embrace of classical rules of design lies a problem of significant and growing scale; namely, not all sound learning occurs through formal science. Our rules about what shall and shall not be cited and published as science may have become too stringent for our own good.[1]

Dr Williams received consulting fees from B. Braun USA during the year 2010.
[a] Department of Anesthesiology, University of Pittsburgh Medical Center, Liliane S. Kaufmann Building, 3471 Fifth Avenue Suite 910, Pittsburgh, PA 15213, USA
[b] Division of Ambulatory Anesthesia, University of Pittsburgh Medical Center, South Side Hospital, 2000 Mary Street, Pittsburgh, PA 15203, USA
* Corresponding author.
E-mail address: phillipsd4@upmc.edu

Anesthesiology Clin 29 (2011) 213–232
doi:10.1016/j.anclin.2011.04.010
1932-2275/11/$ – see front matter © 2011 Elsevier Inc. All rights reserved.
anesthesiology.theclinics.com

Quality care improvements with regional anesthesia use, as measured by patients, surgeons, and anesthesiologists, were striking findings in early studies; these outcomes are now generally accepted. Regional anesthesia (RA) is accepted to provide significant cost benefit to the facility[2] and cost utility to patients.[3,4]

DEFINITIONS
Anesthetic Definitions

Unless otherwise stated, regional anesthesia refers to spinal anesthesia (SA) and peripheral nerve blockade. General anesthesia (GA) is specified as general anesthesia with volatile anesthetics (GAVA) to highlight the implications of volatile anesthetic use. Total intravenous anesthesia (TIVA) refers to general anesthesia maintenance with propofol, thus distinguishing TIVA from GAVA.

Economic Definitions

The economics of health care requires examination of the cost effectiveness of a delivery model (specifically, acute pain management in this review). The model should incorporate cost benefit, cost utility, and the provider interventions.[5]

Cost benefit is one element in the cost-effectiveness calculation. The cost-benefit equation examines the monetary benefits associated with an intervention. The equation, therefore, assumes that a monetary value be used as both the numerator and the denominator. Cost-benefit analysis informs the hospital or medical provider regarding the economic benefit of certain health care delivery models to their institution or practice. Part of the objective in applying this equation is to demonstrate that a cost benefit can be seen with the use of an RA technique, for example, in the ambulatory surgical setting.[2,6]

Cost-utility analysis provides the analyst with a means to incorporate patient-reported benefits that translate to quality of life. Validated outcome measures, such as the Quality of Recovery scale,[7,8] allow patients to determine the health factors that are most pertinent and provides relevant data for this type of analysis.[5] However, in ambulatory RA, other health status surveys can assess patient outcome quality with less respondent burden.[9] Cost utility becomes an increasingly important variable as patients play a greater role in their health care.

ANESTHESIOLOGISTS' IMPACT ON COST

Anesthesiologists play a significant role by selecting interventions that have an impact on cost analysis.[5] The anesthetic plan can significantly affect both cost-benefit and cost-utility calculations.[5,6] Although anesthetic agents have their own associated acquisition costs, downstream cost savings becomes the centerpiece of analysis via patient care streamlining, with both same-day discharge and bypass of the traditional postanesthesia care unit (PACU).[2,10,11]

Given the current political, economic, and social drive to reduce costs while improving the quality and availability of health care, it is prudent to evaluate practices that are shown to deliver the optimum cost-utility (patient-centered) and cost-benefit (hospital-centered) quality care to patients. However, optimum is not always maximum. This point becomes apparent as more procedures are done on an outpatient basis, and our goals as practitioners are to maximize positive outcomes and minimize both adverse effects and costs to the extent feasible. Outpatient procedures eliminate costly services associated with an inpatient stay, such as monitoring, nursing care, laboratory fees, housekeeping and nutrition charges, and so forth.[12]

Anesthesia care safety and effectiveness are at the core of a successful ambulatory surgery model that optimizes cost benefit for the facility and cost utility for patients. Furthermore, subspecialty services, such as ambulatory RA, must be performed on a large enough scale (with sufficient frequency or proportion within an overall case-load) to appreciate real-world cost reduction, for example, in the realm of reliable PACU bypass.[2,13]

Volatile Anesthetics Decrease Cost Utility and Cost Benefit

In same-day orthopedic contexts, a high incidence of unplanned admissions and readmissions for uncontrolled postoperative pain can be common.[14] In various studies comparing GAVA and RA in orthopedic outpatient surgery, a significant differ-ence exists when evaluating the cost of (1) delivering anesthesia, (2) operating room (OR) and PACU time, and (3) necessary postoperative interventions.[2,10,15–18]

The equipment and anesthetic agents required vary significantly between GA and RA. GA most commonly involves the use of instruments to manipulate and secure the airway and the use of volatile agents (GAVA). Although the cost of volatile agents themselves can be significant, it is their side effects that contribute to increased facility costs. Volatile anesthetics are emetogenic[19] and cause transient hyperalgesia.[20,21] In an editorial by Flood (2010),[22] the culturally unpopular declaration is made that the hyperalgesic side effects of volatile agents undermine core elements of our specialty's mission, based on the RCT by Cheng and colleagues[20] (2008) and Tan and colleagues[21] (2010).

In addition to volatile agent-induced hyperalgesia, as well as postoperative nausea and vomiting (PONV),[19] volatile agents increase the need for opioid administration in the PACU after orthopedic surgery in patients to be admitted.[23] In addition, the use of GAVA, airway instrumentation, and opioids does not reduce PACU nursing interven-tions when PACU bypass criteria are used.[24] Furthermore, there is evidence that the use of GAVA leads to higher hospital costs (via forced PACU stays instead of PACU bypass) and unplanned hospital admissions.[2] Overall, the anesthetic medication costs appear to be a minor contributor to overall costs to the facility.[25] However, avoiding GAVA has been shown to result in the reduced cost of anesthesia delivered.[23] In a study by Gonano and colleagues[23] (2006), 40 patients undergoing total hip or total knee arthroplasty were randomized to receive either GAVA or SA; the total cost per case (without accounting for hospital personnel costs) was almost half in the SA group compared to the GAVA group (regardless of volatile agent used). This cost savings was the result of lower overall costs for anesthesia and for recovery. Gonano and colleagues[26] later studied the economic aspects of interscalene block (ISB) versus GAVA (sevoflurane) for arthroscopic shoulder surgery; 40 patients received either GAVA or ISB. The investigators found that cost of anesthesia was lower for ISB. Personnel costs were not included in this study.[26] These studies by Gonano and colleageus[23,26] replicate and further authenticate the clinical reality studies from the previous decade.[15,16]

To summarize, RA by itself, via PACU bypass and shorter PACU lengths of stay, is unlikely to maximize the cost benefit (hospital) and cost utility (patient) to real-world analyses until GAVA is relegated to either legacy status or restricted for use in emer-gencies (or when anesthesia maintenance with propofol [TIVA] is not safely achievable from a hemodynamic standpoint).

Overview of RA Cost Benefits

With propofol use instead of GAVA, reductions in postoperative nausea or vomiting are beneficial to patients.[19,27] The use of RA instead of GAVA helps reduce PONV, pain, and the need for postoperative intravenous opioids.[2,6,18,28–34] Ultimately, PACU length of stay is reduced (if not eliminated).

Reductions in PACU use, including via PACU bypass, lead to hospitals' cost benefit, including reduced postoperative nursing interventions,[2,18,35] reduced unanticipated admissions,[2,36] and faster discharge times.[10,33,34,37–40] Other cost-benefit manifestations to the hospital include reduction in operating room time without an increase in turnover time[17] and reduced cost of anesthesia delivered by avoiding volatile anesthetics.[15,16]

Reduced operating room times

Included in the economic aspects of anesthesia are the costs associated with anesthesia-related use of OR time. In addition to surgical time, operating room time is comprised of anesthesia-controlled time (ACT) and turnover time (TOT). ACT is defined as the time from when patients enter the operating room until readiness for positioning, plus the time from the end of surgery until patients leave the operating room.[17] Induction and recovery from GA typically occurs entirely in the OR and forces an increase in ACT. However, RA can be performed either in the operating room or in a separate preoperative block area. Potential cost benefit (ie, for the hospital) exists in reducing costly operating room time directly related to the delivery of anesthesia. TOT cannot be controlled solely (if at all) by the anesthesia providers[17]; there are additional factors, such as time needed for janitorial staff to clean the OR and time needed by the OR staff to set up for the next case.[41] Anesthesiologists can reduce costly operating room time use by reducing ACT. Cost savings for a hospital can be obtained by the induction of RA in a block area, provided this allows for overall staff reduction or reassigning staff to other value-added activities.[17]

PONV avoidance

Patients commonly experience pain and PONV in the PACU. Retrospective case analysis and RCT have been performed, commonly in orthopedic surgery, to examine the difference in outcomes between GAVA and RA. However, other surgical patient populations have also been studied. One of many illustrations of this involved the comparison of GAVA and RA with paravertebral nerve blocks (PVB) in patients undergoing inguinal hernia repair, in which Hadzic and colleagues[40] found that the patients receiving PVB had less PONV, sore throat, and pain requiring treatment in the first 24 hours.

PACU bypass, reduced length of stay, same-day discharge

Whether patients are scheduled for same-day discharge or for same-day admission, the facility cost savings is typically related to decreasing hospital length of stay. RA reduces hospital length of stay for same-day discharge patients by allowing them to avoid an expensive phase I (PACU) recovery stay. The PACU has the greatest influence on anesthesia-associated cost reduction in same-day discharge patients.[41] Length-of-stay reduction begins with successful same-day discharge without unplanned admission or readmission,[2,14] and is further enhanced by reducing multiple-day hospitalizations to single days.[12,42,43] The costs of a day of hospitalization are not a trivial matter.[44]

It is common sense to acknowledge that accelerating postoperative inpatient stays for a hospital operating at full capacity would lead to more surgical case capacity because there would be more available inpatient beds to route postoperative patients. To the authors' knowledge, however, such logic is not well supported by detailed prospective literature, and capacity planning is most commonly institution-specific, which may be difficult to generalize, requiring simulation research as performed by investigators, such as Dr Franklin Dexter (www.franklin-dexter.net).

Hadzic and colleagues[37] showed that patients receiving RA had a 79% PACU bypass rate compared with 25% for the GAVA group. These patients also met readiness for discharge criteria earlier, had less pain, and were more satisfied with their care. Other studies support this finding.[2,40,45,46] Boutique RA methods, such as selective (unilateral) spinal anesthetics/analgesia, can also be used to improve efficiency while maintaining effectiveness and patient satisfaction.[47–53]

Reduced postoperative admissions and less pain

RA use in orthopedic surgical procedures results in fewer unplanned admissions. Williams and colleagues[18] examined outpatient knee surgeries and showed when no nerve block was performed, more complex surgery was associated with a 10-fold greater unplanned hospital admission, and use of either a femoral plus sciatic block or femoral block alone was associated with 2.5-fold reduction in unplanned admissions. By reducing adverse outcomes, such as PONV and postoperative pain, the use of RA in one retrospective case series from the late 1990s showed reduction in unplanned hospital admission rates from 17% to 4%. The ability to bypass the PACU was significantly associated with the avoidance of GAVA, the use of a femoral nerve block, and the use of preemptive antiemetics[2,10]; these findings have also been shown in other types of outpatient orthopedic surgery.[29,54]

Earlier discharge

In 2005, Hadzic and colleagues[38] compared the time until discharge readiness (number of minutes from the end of the procedure until ready for discharge) for subjects undergoing open rotator cuff surgery. Subjects were randomized to an interscalene block plus propofol sedation (ISB group) and the control group that received GAVA, fentanyl, midazolam, and rocuronium followed by intraarticular and incisional infiltration with 0.25% bupivacaine. The ISB group was ready for home discharge sooner (123 vs 286 minutes for GAVA; $P<.001$), and had a lower unplanned hospital admission rate (4% vs 25%; $P<.05$).[38] This finding has been demonstrated in other contexts of upper-extremity surgery.[55]

Standardization and safety of PACU bypass protocols

Because PACU bypass leads to hospital cost savings in patients receiving RA, it is important to utilize bypass criteria that accounts for the usual recovery from GA and RA. In a simple example, when using the modified Aldrete scoring system,[56] patients receiving RA often will lose 1 point (on the zero-to-10 scale) for not moving all 4 extremities. The White-Song PACU fast-track criteria[57] were developed for outpatients receiving GA but not RA. The WAKE score (Williams and Kentor, 2011[58]) is an update of the Regional Anesthesia PACU Bypass Criteria (RAPBC),[11] properly adjusted for RA use, while incorporating zero-tolerance criteria (pain, nausea, vomiting, shivering, pruritus, lightheadedness) relevant to all patients receiving anesthesia care. The WAKE score (and the previous RAPBC) allows for PACU bypass regardless of RA, GA, monitored anesthesia care, or relevant combinations. The WAKE score evaluates the same 5 recovery categories as does the Modified Aldrete score in which patients are evaluated and scored on movement, blood pressure, level of consciousness, respiratory effort, and pulse oximetry. As with Aldrete, numerical values of zero, 1, or 2 are given in each category and a total score. With WAKE, a score of at least 8 out of 10 is required to allow for PACU bypass, along with meeting all zero-tolerance criteria. Importantly, the movement category assigns the highest score of 2 to patients purposefully moving at least 1 upper and at least 1 lower extremity.[11,58] Furthermore, respiratory status is assessed by the ability (or lack thereof) to cough. The highest score of 2 is given to patients who can cough on command or involuntarily. A score of 1 is given to patients that can cough involuntarily, but not on command; tachypnea, dyspnea, or apnea is given a score of zero.[11,58] Once a standard and rational PACU bypass scoring system is established, then cost savings (from PACU bypass) is more likely to be maximized.

The safety of PACU bypass in outpatient populations, with appropriate and updated criteria, is reinforced in a prospective multicenter outcomes study by Apfelbaum and colleagues.[59] After 1 month of education for physicians, nurses, and ancillary staff, the investigators observed an improvement in the overall rate of PACU bypass from 16% to 58% (P<.001). Patients' receiving GA had an increase in PACU bypass rate from 0.4% to 31.8% (P<.001). Those who received regional, local, or monitored anesthesia care also had an improvement in PACU bypass rate from 29.1% to 84.2% (P<.001). The patients bypassing the PACU experienced a shorter time to recovery without increased morbidity. In this study, usage of short-acting anesthetics was emphasized. This finding demonstrates the importance of education and cultural change required to effectively implement PACU bypass.

Caveats

Cost savings for a single procedure studied, such as anterior cruciate ligament reconstruction,[2] are unlikely enough to generate significant cost benefit via staffing reduction. Also, managers must weigh costs and time required for anesthesiologists and assisting personnel to place blocks in an RA induction room model. In addition, the savings displayed in such studies needs to be extrapolated to large volumes of outpatient orthopedic procedures[2]; citations in this review clearly demonstrate that the tandem of RA and avoidance of GAVA leads to reliable PACU bypass regardless of the surgical procedure being performed (as long as the procedure is amenable to RA and does not require an intraoperative airway device). It seems logical that the PACU bypass success of RA plus propofol TIVA (with a secured airway) would likely rate somewhere between RA and spontaneous airway, and RA combined with GAVA. To the authors' knowledge, such comparative studies have yet to be performed, although such studies would be difficult to gain ethics committee approval for now that GAVA is both known to be emetogenic *and* hyperalgesic.

Defining GA accurately

In the United States, it is important for billing purposes to correctly differentiate and document monitored anesthesia care from GA. According to the American Society of Anesthesiologists' definition of GA, these patients are not able to be aroused with painful stimuli, will frequently have inadequate spontaneous ventilation, will often require some degree of airway intervention, and cardiovascular function may become impaired.[†] The implications of this definition of GA, with respect to billing procedures, have been described elsewhere.[60]

Logistics of delivery

Designated perioperative RA area can improve efficiency, cost reduction, patient satisfaction, surgeon satisfaction, and safety. Tucker and colleagues[61] provide an in-depth description of such a holding areas, as well as monitoring, block cart supplies, resuscitation equipment utilized in the practice at Duke University.

[†] American Society of Anesthesiologists. ASA Position on Monitored Anesthesia Care. 2008. http://www.asahq.org/publicationsAndServices/sgstoc.htm. Accesssed August 18, 2010.

Team effort
All parties involved in patient care must be on board with RA use for conversion from a GAVA culture to solely RA (with or without GA, and avoiding volatile agents). This conversion will first require education by the anesthesiologist regarding advances and advantages of regional anesthesia/analgesia to surgeons, administrators, nursing, and ancillary staff. Williams and Kentor (2000) published a detailed approach and appropriate initial and long-term goals to this approach using a classic plan-do-check-act method,[62] whereas the same investigators,[6] as well as Kahn and Nelson,[63] describe other successful methods to roll out RA programs.

Should one invest in ultrasonography for RA?
There are common questions that arise when considering the purchase of an ultrasound device for placing nerve blocks or catheters that could contribute to the cost-benefit equation. The questions address whether ultrasound is safer, faster, cheaper, and more efficacious. When asking or answering these questions, it is important to specify for which anatomical area or clinical scenario and for single-shot block versus a perineural catheter.

The American Society of Regional Anesthesia (ASRA) executive summary by Neal and colleagues[64] applied evidence-based medicine tactics to evaluate the ultrasound-guided regional anesthesia (UGRA) literature. The executive panel had 3 categories of interest relating to the use of UGRA: (1) block-related outcomes (ie, onset, duration, and patient satisfaction), (2) process-related outcomes (shorter block performance time), and (3) safety-related outcomes. They applied statements of evidence and grades of recommendations to the topics according to the United States Department of Health and Human Services Agency for Health Care Policy and Research. Although there is evidence from at least one RCT (level of evidence: 1b) that UGRA provides a faster sensory onset and higher surrogate block success rates, no grades of recommendations are made for upper-extremity blocks by ASRA because of the wide variability of the study designs with other studies.[64] Similarly with lower-extremity RA, Neal and colleagues[64] applied a level 1b statement of evidence and grade A recommendations for UGRA over traditional methods of nerve localization for lower-extremity blocks in several categories. The same statement of evidence and recommendations (1b grade A) were given for the time to catheter placement in popliteal and other sciatic nerve block catheters. With truncal blocks, although there was little conclusive research regarding UGRA for truncal blocks (paravertebral nerve blocks-PVB, intercostal, transversus abdominis plane, rectus sheath [RS], and ilioinguinal/iliohypogastric [II/IH] blocks), the executive committee gave a statement of evidence 1b and grade A recommendation for the use of UGRA to place RS blocks as ultrasound may reduce the rate of intraperitoneal needle placement. This same level of evidence and recommendation (1b, grade A) was given to the use of UGRA for II/IH nerve blocks in pediatric populations.[64]

Neuraxial blocks Conclusive studies for the use of ultrasound for neuraxial blocks are also lacking. Neal and colleagues[64] distinguished ultrasound-assisted versus ultrasound-guided RA for neuraxial blocks. They applied a level IIa statement of evidence for the use of UGRA over physical examination methods of identifying the correct intervertebral spaces. However, UGRA was inferior to radiographic-guided methods of interspace identification. Also, UGRA was superior (1b) to other methods for predicting skin-to-epidural space depth. Higher success rates (1b) of epidural placement were realized in trainees compared to when trainees did not utilize ultrasound. Also, fewer attempts were required when performing combined spinal/epidural with UGRA than with traditional methods (1b).

Safety The ASRA executive summary determined that there is no conclusive evidence that UGRA reduces the rate of nerve injury. There was evidence (1a) for reduced vascular punctures, and reduced frequency and degree of hemi-diaphragmatic paralysis. However, according to Neal and colleagues,[64] the clinical utility of this evidence is unlikely. Despite the lower volumes of local anesthetics (LA) required for adequate nerve blockade with the use of UGRA (Ia), there is no good evidence (level III) for any reduction in local anesthetic systemic toxicity, nor was there evidence of a reduced rate of pneumothorax (III). Of interest, Matthieu and colleagues[†] demonstrated that a lower LA volume accompanied commonly by UGRA use can come at the expense of a shorter duration of action.[†] Although studies addressing the duration of single-injection nerve blocks are scarce, one should not underdose the duration of a block and risk an unplanned hospital readmission. Hospital readmissions certainly carry their own patient safety risks[65] aside from increased hospital costs.[14]

Is ultrasound cheaper? Liu and John's analysis of the cost of ultrasound-guided nerve blocks showed consistent competitiveness with nerve stimulator as long as a high success rate was maintained using ultrasound.[66] Ultrasound use did not offer favorable cost savings in a hospital setting secondary to a large variety of clinical scenarios.[66] Overall, no conclusive evidence shows UGRA to be inferior to traditional (ie, nerve stimulator) methods of nerve localization.

Inpatient acute pain management

Anesthesiology costs are estimated to be 5.6% for patients having common procedures (appendectomy, cholecystectomy, prostatectomy, discectomy) and scheduled for same-day admission.[25] The operating-room and hospital-ward costs comprise the greatest proportion of total hospital cost. However, it is likely that anesthesiology decisions affect postoperative resource consumption. This area should be the target of future cost-savings research. Existing research by Hebl and colleagues,[67] Ilfeld and colleagues,[12] and Capdevila and colleagues[68] support the inpatient use of RA for reduced length of stay and hospital cost reduction. However, acute pain service staffing and ancillary costs to ensure either cost neutrality (ie, break even) or cost savings are now at the forefront as necessary for future study.

At present, it is difficult to assess the economics of an inpatient acute pain service because the literature is lacking, other than that described by Hebl and colleagues[67] at the Mayo Clinic. The quantity of literature is not the only factor making economic assessments difficult. What constitutes an acute pain service (how it is staffed, how it is underwritten, and what its role is) is not uniform among institutions. Therefore, comparing economic and outcome data between institutions may not be reliable because it is unlikely that acute pain services would be uniform.

According to the American Society of Anesthesiologists' Task Force on Acute Pain Management,[69] an acute pain service should consist of (1) education and training for health care providers, (2) patient outcome monitoring, (3) documentation of monitoring, (4) outcome monitoring at an institutional level, (5) 24-hour anesthesiologist coverage to provide acute pain management, and the (6) employment of a dedicated acute pain service.

For inpatients, several well-designed outcome studies have been published evaluating postoperative analgesia that utilizes epidural catheters.[70–75] If the correct patient

---

† Ponrouch M, Bouic N, Bringuier S, et al. Decreasing local anesthetic volume influences duration of peripheral nerve block but not onset time [abstract]. Proceedings of the 2009 Annual Meeting of the American Society Anesthesiologists.

population is chosen for epidural catheter pain management (namely high-risk patients undergoing major surgery), a favorable cost-benefit ratio results.[73,74]

Outcome data and cost analyses of RA-based acute pain services emphasizing peripheral nerve blocks for inpatients are lacking compared with the literature for epidural models.[70] Obviously, as in epidural research, the peripheral RA studies should identify high-risk patients most likely to benefit from a particular technique.[70]

The application of peripheral RA techniques can likely advance the achievements of an acute pain service by reducing opioid consumption, nursing interventions, and hospital length of stay. Although patient-controlled analgesia (PCA, utilizing intravenous opioids) can reduce the time required by nurses to administer opioids, PCA may not reduce the time that nursing spends on treatment of opioid-related side effects (nausea, vomiting, pruritus, constipation, sedation). It is accepted that peripheral RA techniques are opioid sparing. As a result, we can combine the benefits of opioid sparing and increase the use of patient-controlled perineural catheters, as long as restrictions on patient ambulation are in place, when appropriate (eg, lower-extremity perineural infusions). Patient-controlled analgesia need not be restricted to the self-administering of intravenous opioids in the hospital setting. Opioid sparing, reductions in mechanical ventilation time, and length of stay in the intensive care unit or the hospital are appropriately targeted for cost containment.

To accurately assess what is cost savings and cost benefit for inpatients is challenging. Most of the cited publications on the cost benefit and cost utility of regional anesthesia/analgesia for patients undergoing ambulatory surgery focused on bypassing the PACU for cost savings. Future studies of surgical inpatients should not only evaluate the proven PACU bypass (or reduced length of PACU stay) savings but also the fewer nursing interventions that may result from RA (anesthesia *and* analgesia) throughout the hospital stay. Other high-cost areas for inpatients, such as the intensive care unit, or high-cost therapies, such as ventilator use, should also be a focus of future cost-benefit analyses addressing RA. It is reasonable to assume that reduced ventilator days, intensive care unit days, and total hospital stay traced back to RA use (whether operative or nonoperative) will lead to hospital cost savings. However, the savings can likely be best quantified and maximized by specifically studying those patients most likely to benefit.[70]

Postoperative Infections and Potential Beneficial Role of RA

Surgical site infections (SSI) complicate between 5% and 10% of all surgeries.[76–82] They are estimated to increase hospital length of stay by 48% to 310% and increase cost by 34% to 226% when compared to patients without an SSI.[83] Early seeding of the surgical site is one of the key factors in the formation of SSIs.[84] Therefore, physiologic conditions during this time period and in to the early postoperative period may be critical to the formation of these infections.[78,84,85]

Polymorphonuclear leukocytes (PMN) release oxygen free radicals to kill bacteria. Low blood flow states caused by hypothermia-induced vasoconstriction or sympathetic nervous system response to pain reduce the number of surgical site PMNs and tissue oxygen tension.[86,87] The local tissue oxygen tension is used by PMNs for superoxide radical formation and eventual killing of bacteria.[84] Anesthetic techniques that prevent vasoconstriction at the surgical site (RA and the prevention of hypothermia) may reduce the occurrence of SSIs.[87,88] Prospective, RCT data support the use of RA (specifically thoracic epidural) to increase surgical-site tissue oxygen tension.[86,89] However, more studies are required to support the direct relationship between RA use, specifically related to perineural catheters and SSI prevention. Furthermore, the risks of perineural catheter infections occurring, versus SSIs avoided, will require further elucidation.

Regional Anesthesia and Malignancy

The perioperative period appears to be more important than previously considered for long-term outcomes. This point is true for the prevention of surgical site infections by timely administration of antibiotics and may be true for the prevention of metastasis in oncology patients.[90] Data from the specialties of immunology and oncology report details regarding the body's response to stress (surgical or anesthetic related) of contributing to micrometastasis and subsequent cancer recurrence.[90–95] Specific anesthetics also show evidence of immunosuppression and may contribute to cancer recurrence.[96–98]

The physiologic response to perioperative stress is well documented. Just as in the current investigations of the sympathetic nervous system's contribution to poor molecular oxygen tension at the surgical site, the sympathetic nervous system (as well as surgical manipulation of tumors) may be culpable for metastasis during surgery.[99] The specific immune mechanism appears to be the suppression of natural killer (NK) cell activity, which correlates with a higher mortality in colorectal,[100,101] gastric,[102] lung,[103] and head and neck malignancies.[104,105]

Medications often administered during an isolated general anesthetic, such as opioids (morphine specifically), ketamine, pentothal, and volatile agents, are shown to have some inhibitory effect on cell-mediated immunity (NK cells), the most important defense against malignancies.[90,96–98] The clinical implications of anesthesia-related immunosuppression is unclear.

Retrospective RA data by Exadaktylos and colleagues,[106] Biki and colleagues,[107] and Christopherson and colleagues[108] show an association between the use of RA techniques and reduced cancer recurrence. There is also early evidence that avoidance of GAVA may be beneficial.[109] A more recent retrospective study by Wuethrich and colleagues[110] showed an association between GAVA plus thoracic epidural analgesia use (compared with no epidural) and reduced clinical progression of prostate cancer. The authors of that study defined clinical progression as radiologic evidence of recurrence or metastatic disease. The same study showed no difference in overall survival or biochemical recurrence. Therefore, no data are conclusive regarding anesthetic technique on cancer recurrence, but it is hoped that future and ongoing[111] studies will answer these questions.

Although the economics of cancer recurrence is difficult to quantify, it is likely to be extremely large. Assuming that cancer recurrence costs are vast, then preventing even a small percentage of metastases and recurrence would have a tremendous impact on cost benefit and cost utility. In fact, a recent cost analysis addressing breast cancer screening and diagnosis reported that the median cost per screening is approximately $100, whereas the median costs of diagnosis is approximately $10,000.[112] The costs of treatment notwithstanding, it follows that the costs of diagnosing and treating a cancer recurrence far exceed the costs of screening (for recurrence), and if RA use proves to be central to the prevention of cancer recurrence, then this public health responsibility should not be taken lightly.

Reduced blood transfusions

Many RCT evaluating the effect of RA on surgical blood loss and reduced blood product transmission have been published specifically addressing total joint arthroplasty utilizing epidural or spinal anesthesia.[113–115] Most data support the use of RA (spinal or epidural) to reduce surgical blood loss in hip arthroplasty. In a meta-analysis by Guay,[116] evidence showed that spinal anesthesia reduced surgical blood loss, but did **not** reduce the number of patients transfused. However, Rashiq and Finnegan[117] retrospectively analyzed (n = 1875) patients who received neuraxial anesthesia hip and knee arthroplasty, and found a reduced risk for blood transfusion in hip arthroplasty but not for knee arthroplasty. Furthermore, when comparing GAVA with a lumbar plexus block with GAVA alone, Stevens and colleagues[118] found a reduced blood loss with the GAVA with lumbar plexus block group after total hip arthroplasty, although this was this study's secondary endpoint. Finally, Chelly and colleagues[119] reported (as a secondary outcome) less blood loss after total knee replacement with the use of continuous femoral perineural infusions (when compared with epidural local anesthetic or intravenous opioid patient-controlled analgesia).

Regarding the cost of transfusions, there were approximately 30 million blood products transfused in the United States in 2006.[‡] According to Goodnough and colleagues,[120,121] the rate of red cell transfusion has been decreasing since a peak transfusion rate occurred in 1986.[120,121] Despite these trends, blood product transfusion is expensive. Although the typical acquisition cost of 1 unit of packed red blood cells (PRBCs) can be priced as low as less than $200/unit (Jonathan Waters, MD, personal communication, March 24, 2010), PRBCs administered to surgical patients is estimated to have a median cost between $500 and $1200, when incorporating all the activity-based costs into the complex process of blood banking.[122] Certainly, any adverse effects of blood product transfusion, such as disease transmission, transfusion-related lung injury, immunosuppression, allergic reactions, mismatch errors, coagulopathy, hypothermia, and so forth, incur their own added costs. This reduction in transfusion requirements with regional anesthesia has to be reconsidered in the climate of blood-conservation programs for various surgical procedures.

Societal Cost of Poor Pain Management

The presence of preoperative pain and poorly controlled acute postoperative pain are demonstrated to be risk factors for chronic postsurgical pain (CPSP) development.[123–130] The highest incidence of chronic postoperative pain occurs with (1) limb amputation (30% –81%), (2) thoracotomy (50%), (3) breast surgery (11%–57%), (4) cholecystectomy (3%–56%), and (5) inguinal hernia repair (11.5%).[131]

Data aimed at the prevention of CPSP are controversial. Research by Obata and colleagues[132] support the use of preemptive thoracic epidural for a reduction in post-thoracotomy syndrome. The American Association of Anesthesiologists' Practice Guidelines for Acute Pain Management in the Perioperative Setting only support improved perioperative pain control with RA techniques, rather than explicitly assuming RA use to lead to reduced CPSP.[69] However, because poorly controlled perioperative pain predicts the development of CPSP, then the use of RA techniques for superior postoperative pain management seems to be an appropriate target for ongoing research, both prospective and retrospective.

Few data investigate the cost of poorly controlled acute postoperative pain. The total cost of this failure to treat would likely be (1) the sum of the necessary interventions aimed at responding to the acute pain; (2) the missed cost savings if RA would have been appropriate (cost of increased length of stay, readmissions, nursing interventions, and so forth), and (3) the long-term costs of a chronic pain condition. These long-term costs include poor work productivity or absenteeism, and disability payments.[133]

---

‡ Available at: http://www.aabb.org/resources/bct/pages/bloodfaq.aspx#a1. Accessed August 24, 2010.

Interestingly, Stewart and colleagues[134] published a cross-sectional study showing that poor productivity after returning to work (in patients with common chronic pain conditions) incurs the most economic burden on society (as opposed to absenteeism). Therefore, cost savings appears not to be in returning patients to work, but in returning patients to productive work through the primary prevention of chronic pain development. It is also unclear what percentage of patients with chronic pain is from the CPSP subgroup. More data are needed regarding the impact of RA both on CPSP and on the economic burden to patients, hospitals, and society.

SUMMARY

Research from the last 2 decades confirms that outpatient RA is accepted to provide significant cost benefit to the facility and cost utility to patients. Although there is less inpatient research regarding the cost benefit and cost utility of RA, the outcomes appear similar. More inpatient RA research is needed to make this conclusion. However, the cost benefit and cost utility of: (1) PACU bypass, (2) reduced nursing time spent on opioid and GAVA side effects, (3) reduced hospital and intensive care unit stay, and (4) reduced ventilator days must be included in the cost analyses to expose the financial benefits of RA. Future financial analyses of acute pain services may prove to be more difficult because of varying patterns of practices (including staffing). Prior to making conclusions on the cost benefit and cost utility of an inpatient acute pain service, one should compare research between institutions in which the roles of the services are comparable. The evidence for ultrasound-guided (and ultrasound-assisted) RA shows that UGRA is not inferior to traditional methods (most often peripheral nerve stimulation) and is superior in certain scenarios previously described. Furthermore, the cost of UGRA is comparable to peripheral nerve stimulator (PNS)-guided nerve blocks in outpatients, but does not appear to be so for inpatients.

It is difficult to ignore the mounting evidence against the use of GAVA in the subspecialty contexts of cancer surgery, surgery leading to blood transfusion, preventing surgical site infections, and chronic postsurgical pain. Evolving evidence for RA superiority in some of these areas, and suggestive evidence in others, brings a new outlook both for anesthesiology as a subspecialty of medicine and RA as a key component of the practice of acute pain medicine. Over time, these evolving concepts at present may lead to RA use in the future becoming the rule rather than the exception.

REFERENCES

1. Berwick DM. Harvesting knowledge from improvement. JAMA 1996;275:877.
2. Williams BA, Kentor ML, Vogt MT, et al. The economics of nerve block pain management after anterior cruciate ligament reconstruction: Significant hospital cost savings via associated PACU bypass and same-day discharge. Anesthesiology 2004;100:697.
3. Ilfeld BM, Meyer RS, Le LT, et al. Health-related quality of life after tricompartment knee arthroplasty with and without an extended-duration continuous femoral nerve block: a prospective, 1-year follow-up of a randomized, triple-masked, placebo-controlled study. Anesth Analg 2009;108:1320.
4. Ilfeld BM, Ball ST, Gearen PF, et al. Health-related quality of life after hip arthroplasty with and without an extended-duration continuous posterior lumbar plexus nerve block: a prospective, 1-year follow-up of a randomized, triple-masked, placebo-controlled study. Anesth Analg 2009;109:586.

5. Williams BA, Kentor ML, Chelly JE. Cost-benefit and cost-utility analyses: outpatient implications. In: Steele SM, Nielsen KC, Klein SM, editors. Ambulatory anesthesia and perioperative analgesia. 1st edition. New York: McGraw-Hill; 2004. p. 135–44.
6. Williams BA, Kentor ML. Making an ambulatory surgery center suitable for regional anaesthesia. Bailliere's Best Pract Res Clin Anaesthesiol 2002;16:175.
7. Myles PS, Hunt JO, Nightingale CE, et al. Development and psychometric testing of a Quality of Recovery score after general anesthesia and surgery in adults. Anesth Analg 1999;88:83.
8. Myles PS, Weitkamp B, Jones K, et al. Validity and reliability of a postoperative quality of recovery score: the QoR-40. Br J Anaesth 2000;84:11.
9. Bost JE, Williams BA, Bottegal MT, et al. The 8-Item Short-Form Health Survey and the physical comfort composite score of the quality of recovery 40-item Scale provide the most responsive assessments of pain, physical function, and mental function during the first 4 days after ambulatory knee surgery with regional anesthesia. Anesth Analg 2007;105:1693.
10. Williams BA, Kentor ML, Williams JP, et al. PACU bypass after outpatient knee surgery is associated with fewer unplanned hospital admissions but more phase II nursing interventions. Anesthesiology 2002;97:981.
11. Williams BA. For outpatients, does regional anesthesia truly shorten the hospital stay, and how should we define postanesthesia care unit bypass eligibility? Anesthesiology 2004;101:3.
12. Ilfeld BM, Mariano ER, Williams BA, et al. Hospitalization costs of total knee arthroplasty with a continuous femoral nerve block provided only in the hospital versus on an ambulatory basis: a retrospective, case-control, cost-minimization analysis. Reg Anesth Pain Med 2007;32:46.
13. Dexter F, Tinker JH. Analysis of strategies to decrease postanesthesia care unit costs [see comments]. Anesthesiology 1995;82:94.
14. Coley KC, Williams BA, DaPos SV, et al. Retrospective evaluation of unanticipated admissions and readmissions after same day surgery and associated costs. J Clin Anesth 2002;14:349.
15. Williams BA, DeRiso BM, Engel LB, et al. Benchmarking the perioperative process: II. Introducing anesthesia clinical pathways to improve processes and outcomes, and reduce nursing labor intensity in ambulatory orthopedic surgery. J Clin Anesth 1998;10:561.
16. Williams BA, DeRiso BM, Figallo CM, et al. Benchmarking the perioperative process: III. Effects of regional anesthesia clinical pathway techniques on process efficiency and recovery profiles in ambulatory orthopedic surgery. J Clin Anesth 1998;10:570.
17. Williams BA, Kentor ML, Williams JP, et al. Process analysis in outpatient knee surgery: Effects of regional and general anesthesia on anesthesia-controlled time. Anesthesiology 2000;93:529.
18. Williams BA, Kentor ML, Vogt MT, et al. Femoral-sciatic nerve blocks for complex outpatient knee surgery are associated with less postoperative pain before same-day discharge: a review of 1200 consecutive cases from the period 1996–1999. Anesthesiology 2003;98:1206.
19. Apfel CC, Korttila K, Abdalla M, et al. A factorial trial of six interventions for the prevention of postoperative nausea and vomiting. N Engl J Med 2004;350:2441.
20. Cheng SS, Yeh J, Flood P. Anesthesia matters: patients anesthetized with propofol have less postoperative pain than those anesthetized with isoflurane. Anesth Analg 2008;106:264.

21. Tan T, Bhinder R, Carey M, et al. Day-surgery patients anesthetized with propofol have less postoperative pain than those anesthetized with sevoflurane. Anesth Analg 2010;111:83.
22. Flood P. PRO: accumulating evidence for an outrageous claim. Anesth Analg 2010;111:86.
23. Gonano C, Leitgeb U, Sitzwohl C, et al. Spinal versus general anesthesia for orthopedic surgery: anesthesia drug and supply costs. Anesth Analg 2006; 102:524.
24. Song D, Chung F, Ronayne M, et al. Fast-tracking (bypassing the PACU) does not reduce nursing workload after ambulatory surgery. Br J Anaesth 2004;93:768.
25. Macario A, Vitez TS, Dunn B, et al. Where are the costs in perioperative care? Analysis of hospital costs and charges for inpatient surgical care [see comments]. Anesthesiology 1995;83:1138.
26. Gonano C, Kettner SC, Ernstbrunner M, et al. Comparison of economical aspects of interscalene brachial plexus blockade and general anaesthesia for arthroscopic shoulder surgery. Br J Anaesth 2009;103:428.
27. Sneyd JR, Carr A, Byrom WD, et al. A meta-analysis of nausea and vomiting following maintenance of anaesthesia with propofol or inhalational agents. Eur J Anaesthesiol 1998;15:433.
28. Borgeat A, Ekatodramis G, Schenker CA. Postoperative nausea and vomiting in regional anesthesia: a review. Anesthesiology 2003;98:530.
29. Kentor ML, Williams BA. Antiemetics in outpatient regional anesthesia for invasive orthopedic surgery. Int Anesthesiol Clin 2005;43:197.
30. Williams BA, Kentor ML, Vogt MT, et al. Reduction of verbal pain scores after anterior cruciate ligament reconstruction with two-day continuous femoral nerve block: a randomized clinical trial. Anesthesiology 2006;104:315.
31. Williams BA, Kentor ML, Irrgang JJ, et al. Nausea, vomiting, sleep, and restfulness upon discharge home after outpatient anterior cruciate ligament reconstruction with regional anesthesia and multimodal analgesia/antiemesis. Reg Anesth Pain Med 2007;32:193.
32. Skledar SJ, Williams BA, Vallejo MC, et al. Eliminating postoperative nausea and vomiting in outpatient surgery with multimodal strategies including low doses of nonsedating, off-patent antiemetics: is "zero tolerance" achievable? ScientificWorldJournal 2007;7:959.
33. Pavlin DJ, Chen C, Penaloza DA, et al. Pain as a factor complicating recovery and discharge after ambulatory surgery. Anesth Analg 2002;95:627.
34. Pavlin DJ, Rapp SE, Polissar NL, et al. Factors affecting discharge time in adult outpatients. Anesth Analg 1998;87:816.
35. Kitz DS, McCartney M, Kissick JF, et al. Examining nursing personnel costs: controlled versus noncontrolled oral analgesic agents. J Nurs Adm 1989;19:10.
36. White PF, Issioui T, Skrivanek GD, et al. The use of a continuous popliteal sciatic nerve block after surgery involving the foot and ankle: does it improve the quality of recovery? Anesth Analg 2003;97:1303.
37. Hadzic A, Arliss J, Kerimoglu B, et al. A comparison of infraclavicular nerve block versus general anesthesia for hand and wrist surgery in day-case surgery. Anesthesiology 2004;101:127.
38. Hadzic A, Williams BA, Karaca PE, et al. For outpatient rotator cuff surgery, nerve block anesthesia provides superior same-day recovery over general anesthesia. Anesthesiology 2005;102:1001.

39. Hadzic A, Karaca PE, Hobeika P, et al. Peripheral nerve blocks result in superior recovery profile compared with general anesthesia in outpatient knee arthroscopy. Anesth Analg 2005;100:976.

40. Hadzic A, Kerimoglu B, Loreio D, et al. Paravertebral blocks provide superior same-day recovery over general anesthesia for patients undergoing inguinal hernia repair. Anesth Analg 2006;102:1076.

41. Williams BA, Motolenich P, Kentor ML. Hospital facilities and resource management: economic impact of a high-volume regional anesthesia program for outpatients. Int Anesthesiol Clin 2005;43:43.

42. Ilfeld BM, Le LT, Meyer RS, et al. Ambulatory continuous femoral nerve blocks decrease time to discharge readiness after tricompartment total knee arthroplasty: a randomized, triple-masked, placebo-controlled study. Anesthesiology 2008;108:703.

43. Ilfeld BM, Vandenborne K, Duncan PW, et al. Ambulatory continuous interscalene nerve blocks decrease the time to discharge readiness after total shoulder arthroplasty: a randomized, triple-masked, placebo-controlled study. Anesthesiology 2006;105:999.

44. Woolhandler S, Himmelstein DU. Costs of care and administration at for-profit and other hospitals in the United States. N Engl J Med 1997;336:769.

45. Chan VW, Peng PW, Kaszas Z, et al. A comparative study of general anesthesia, intravenous regional anesthesia, and axillary block for outpatient hand surgery: clinical outcome and cost analysis. Anesth Analg 2001;93:1181.

46. Singelyn FJ, Lhotel L, Fabre B. Pain relief after arthroscopic shoulder surgery: a comparison of intraarticular analgesia, suprascapular nerve block, and interscalene brachial plexus block. Anesth Analg 2004;99:589.

47. Borghi B, Stagni F, Bugamelli S, et al. Unilateral spinal block for outpatient knee arthroscopy: a dose-finding study. J Clin Anesth 2003;15:351.

48. Casati A, Fanelli G. Unilateral spinal anesthesia. State of the art. Minerva Anestesiol 2001;67:855.

49. Fanelli G, Borghi B, Casati A, et al. Unilateral bupivacaine spinal anesthesia for outpatient knee arthroscopy. Italian Study Group on Unilateral Spinal Anesthesia. Can J Anaesth 2000;47:746.

50. Casati A, Fanelli G, Beccaria P, et al. Block distribution and cardiovascular effects of unilateral spinal anaesthesia by 0.5% hyperbaric bupivacaine. A clinical comparison with bilateral spinal block. Minerva Anestesiol 1998;64:307.

51. Casati A, Coppelleri G, Fanelli G. Unilateral spinal anesthesia: fact or fiction? Reg Anesth 1997;22:594.

52. Casati A, Fanelli G. Restricting spinal block to the operative side: why not? Reg Anesth Pain Med 2004;29:4.

53. Esmaoglu A, Karaoglu S, Mizrak A, et al. Bilateral vs. unilateral spinal anesthesia for outpatient knee arthroscopies. Knee Surg Sports Traumatol Arthrosc 2004; 12:155.

54. Williams BA, Kentor ML. Fast-track ambulatory anesthesia: impact on nursing workload when analgesia and antiemetic prophylaxis are near-optimal. Can J Anaesth 2007;54:243.

55. Gebhard RE, Al-Samsam T, Greger J, et al. Distal nerve blocks at the wrist for outpatient carpal tunnel surgery offer intraoperative cardiovascular stability and reduce discharge time. Anesth Analg 2002;95:351.

56. Aldrete JA. The post-anesthesia recovery score revisited. J Clin Anesth 1995; 7:89.

57. White PF, Song D. New criteria for fast-tracking after outpatient anesthesia: a comparison with the modified Aldrete's scoring system. Anesth Analg 1999; 88:1069.
58. Williams BA, Kentor ML. The "WAKE Score". Int Anesthesiol Clin 2011;49(3).
59. Apfelbaum JL, Walawander CA, Grasela TH, et al. Eliminating intensive postoperative care in same-day surgery patients using short-acting anesthetics. Anesthesiology 2002;97(1):66–74.
60. Greger J, Williams BA. Billing for outpatient regional anesthesia services in the United States. Int Anesthesiol Clin 2005;43:33.
61. Tucker MS, Nielsen KC, Steele SM. Nerve block induction rooms–physical plant setup, monitoring equipment, block cart, and resuscitation cart. Int Anesthesiol Clin 2005;43:55.
62. Williams BA, Kentor ML. Clinical pathways and the anesthesiologist. Current Anesthesiology Reports 2000;2:418.
63. Kahn RL, Nelson DA. Regional anesthesia group practice in multihospital private practice settings and in orthopedic specialty hospitals. Int Anesthesiol Clin 2005;43:15.
64. Neal JM, Brull R, Chan VW, et al. The ASRA evidence-based medicine assessment of ultrasound-guided regional anesthesia and pain medicine: executive summary. Reg Anesth Pain Med 2010;35:S1.
65. Williams BA, Sakai T. Complications that can arise in orthopedic patients when regional anesthesia is not used. In: Atlee JL, editor. Complications in Anesthesia. 2nd edition. Philadelphia: Elsevier; 2006. p. 265–8.
66. Liu SS, John RS. Modeling cost of ultrasound versus nerve stimulator guidance for nerve blocks with sensitivity analysis. Reg Anesth Pain Med 2010;35:57.
67. Hebl JR, Dilger JA, Byer DE, et al. A pre-emptive multimodal pathway featuring peripheral nerve block improves perioperative outcomes after major orthopedic surgery. Reg Anesth Pain Med 2008;33:510.
68. Capdevila X, Barthelet Y, Biboulet P, et al. Effects of perioperative analgesic technique on the surgical outcome and duration of rehabilitation after major knee surgery. Anesthesiology 1999;91:8.
69. American Society of Anesthesiologists Task Force on Acute Pain M, American Society of Anesthesiologists Task Force on Acute Pain M. Practice guidelines for acute pain management in the perioperative setting: an updated report by the American Society of Anesthesiologists Task Force on Acute Pain Management. Anesthesiology 2004;100:1573.
70. Rauck RL. Cost-effectiveness and cost/benefit ratio of acute pain management. Regional Anesthesia 1996;21:139.
71. Liu SS, Carpenter RL, Mackey DC, et al. Effects of perioperative analgesic technique on rate of recovery after colon surgery. Anesthesiology 1995;83:757.
72. Christopherson R, Beattie C, Frank SM, et al. Perioperative morbidity in patients randomized to epidural or general anesthesia for lower extremity vascular surgery. Perioperative Ischemia Randomized Anesthesia Trial Study Group. Anesthesiology 1993;79:422.
73. Tuman KJ, McCarthy RJ, March RJ, et al. Effects of epidural anesthesia and analgesia on coagulation and outcome after major vascular surgery. Anesth Analg 1991;73:696.
74. Yeager MP, Glass DD, Neff RK, et al. Epidural anesthesia and analgesia in high-risk surgical patients. Anesthesiology 1987;66:729.
75. Rawal N, Sjostrand U, Christoffersson E, et al. Comparison of intramuscular and epidural morphine for postoperative analgesia in the grossly obese:

influence on postoperative ambulation and pulmonary function. Anesth Analg 1984;63:583.

76. Taylor EW, Byrne DJ, Leaper DJ, et al. Antibiotic prophylaxis and open groin hernia repair. World J Surg 1997;21:811.

77. Lizan-Garcia M, Garcia-Caballero J, Asensio-Vegas A, et al. Risk factors for surgical-wound infection in general surgery: a prospective study. Infect Control Hosp Epidemiol 1997;18:310.

78. Kurz A, Sessler DI, Lenhardt R, et al. Perioperative normothermia to reduce the incidence of surgical-wound infection and shorten hospitalization. Study of Wound Infection and Temperature Group. N Engl J Med 1996;334:1209.

79. Keeling NJ, Morgan MW, Keeling NJ, et al. Inpatient and post-discharge wound infections in general surgery. Ann R Coll Surg Engl 1995;77:245.

80. Bailey IS, Karran SE, Toyn K, et al. Community surveillance of complications after hernia surgery. BMJ 1992;304:469 [Erratum appears in BMJ 1992; 304(6829):739].

81. Law DJ, Mishriki SF, Jeffery PJ, et al. The importance of surveillance after discharge from hospital in the diagnosis of postoperative wound infection. Ann R Coll Surg Engl 1990;72:207.

82. Bremmelgaard A, Raahave D, Beier-Holgersen R, et al. Computer-aided surveillance of surgical infections and identification of risk factors. J Hosp Infect 1989;13:1.

83. Broex EC, van Asselt AD, Bruggeman CA, et al. Surgical site infections: how high are the costs? J Hosp Infect 2009;72:193.

84. Miles AA, Miles EM, Burke J, et al. The value and duration of defense reactions of the skin to the primary lodgment of bacteria. Br J Exp Pathol 1957;38:79.

85. Melling AC, Ali B, Scott EM, et al. Effects of preoperative warming on the incidence of wound infection after clean surgery: a randomised controlled trial. Lancet 2001;358:876 [Erratum appears in Lancet 2002;359(9309):896].

86. Kabon B, Fleischmann E, Treschan T, et al. Thoracic epidural anesthesia increases tissue oxygenation during major abdominal surgery. Anesth Analg 1812;97:2003.

87. Sessler DI. Neuraxial anesthesia and surgical site infection. Anesthesiology 2010;113:265.

88. Chang CC, Lin HC, Lin HW, et al. Anesthetic management and surgical site infections in total hip or knee replacement: a population-based study. Anesthesiology 2010;113:279.

89. Buggy DJ, Doherty WL, Hart EM, et al. Postoperative wound oxygen tension with epidural or intravenous analgesia: a prospective, randomized, single-blind clinical trial. Anesthesiology 2002;97:952.

90. Ben-Eliyahu S, Ben-Eliyahu S. The promotion of tumor metastasis by surgery and stress: immunological basis and implications for psychoneuroimmunology. Brain Behav Immun 2003;17(Suppl 1):S27.

91. Goldfarb Y, Ben-Eliyahu S, Goldfarb Y, et al. Surgery as a risk factor for breast cancer recurrence and metastasis: mediating mechanisms and clinical prophylactic approaches. Breast Dis 2006;26:99.

92. Demicheli R, Miceli R, Moliterni A, et al. Breast cancer recurrence dynamics following adjuvant CMF is consistent with tumor dormancy and mastectomy-driven acceleration of the metastatic process. Ann Oncol 2005;16:1449.

93. Yamashita JI, Kurusu Y, Fujino N, et al. Detection of circulating tumor cells in patients with non-small cell lung cancer undergoing lobectomy by video-assisted thoracic surgery: a potential hazard for intraoperative hematogenous tumor cell dissemination. J Thorac Cardiovasc Surg 2000;119:899.

94. Denis MG, Lipart C, Leborgne J, et al. Detection of disseminated tumor cells in peripheral blood of colorectal cancer patients. Int J Cancer 1997;74:540.

95. Eschwege P, Dumas F, Blanchet P, et al. Haematogenous dissemination of prostatic epithelial cells during radical prostatectomy. Lancet 1995;346:1528.

96. Sacerdote P, Bianchi M, Gaspani L, et al. The effects of tramadol and morphine on immune responses and pain after surgery in cancer patients. Anesth Analg 2000;90:1411.

97. Brand JM, Kirchner H, Poppe C, et al. The effects of general anesthesia on human peripheral immune cell distribution and cytokine production. Clin Immunol Immunopathol 1997;83:190.

98. Markovic SN, Knight PR, Murasko DM, et al. Inhibition of interferon stimulation of natural killer cell activity in mice anesthetized with halothane or isoflurane. Anesthesiology 1993;78:700.

99. Melamed R, Rosenne E, Shakhar K, et al. Marginating pulmonary-NK activity and resistance to experimental tumor metastasis: suppression by surgery and the prophylactic use of a beta-adrenergic antagonist and a prostaglandin synthesis inhibitor. Brain Behav Immun 2005;19:114.

100. Tartter PI, Steinberg B, Barron DM, et al. The prognostic significance of natural killer cytotoxicity in patients with colorectal cancer. Arch Surg 1987;122:1264.

101. Koda K, Saito N, Takiguchi N, et al. Preoperative natural killer cell activity: correlation with distant metastases in curatively research colorectal carcinomas. Int Surg 1997;82:190.

102. Takeuchi H, Maehara Y, Tokunaga E, et al. Prognostic significance of natural killer cell activity in patients with gastric carcinoma: a multivariate analysis. Am J Gastroenterol 2001;96:574.

103. Fujisawa T, Yamaguchi Y, Fujisawa T, et al. Autologous tumor killing activity as a prognostic factor in primary resected nonsmall cell carcinoma of the lung. Cancer 1997;79:474.

104. Brittenden J, Heys SD, Ross J, et al. Natural killer cells and cancer. Cancer 1996;77:1226.

105. Schantz SP, Savage HE, Racz T, et al. Immunologic determinants of head and neck cancer response to induction chemotherapy. J Clin Oncol 1989;7:857.

106. Exadaktylos AK, Buggy DJ, Moriarty DC, et al. Can anesthetic technique for primary breast cancer surgery affect recurrence or metastasis? Anesthesiology 2006;105:660.

107. Biki B, Mascha E, Moriarty DC, et al. Anesthetic technique for radical prostatectomy surgery affects cancer recurrence: a retrospective analysis. Anesthesiology 2008;109:180.

108. Christopherson R, James KE, Tableman M, et al. Long-term survival after colon cancer surgery: a variation associated with choice of anesthesia. Anesth Analg 2008;107:325.

109. Schlagenhauff B, Ellwanger U, Breuninger H, et al. Prognostic impact of the type of anaesthesia used during the excision of primary cutaneous melanoma. Melanoma Res 2000;10:165.

110. Wuethrich PY, Hsu Schmitz SF, Kessler TM, et al. Potential influence of the anesthetic technique used during open radical prostatectomy on prostate cancer-related outcome: a retrospective study. Anesthesiology 2010;113(3):570–6.

111. Sessler DI, Ben-Eliyahu S, Mascha EJ, et al. Can regional analgesia reduce the risk of recurrence after breast cancer? methodology of a multicenter randomized trial. Contemp Clin Trials 2008;29:517.

112. Ekwueme DU, Gardner JG, Subramanian S, et al. Cost analysis of the National Breast and Cervical Cancer Early Detection Program: selected states, 2003 to 2004. Cancer 2008;112:626.
113. Borghi B, Casati A, Iuorio S, et al. Frequency of hypotension and bradycardia during general anesthesia, epidural anesthesia, or integrated epidural-general anesthesia for total hip replacement. J Clin Anesth 2002;14:102.
114. Dauphin A, Raymer KE, Stanton EB, et al. Comparison of general anesthesia with and without lumbar epidural for total hip arthroplasty: effects of epidural block on hip arthroplasty. J Clin Anesth 1997;9:200.
115. Modig J, Karlstrom G, Modig J, et al. Intra- and post-operative blood loss and haemodynamics in total hip replacement when performed under lumbar epidural versus general anaesthesia. Eur J Anaesthesiol 1987;4:345.
116. Guay J, Guay J. The effect of neuraxial blocks on surgical blood loss and blood transfusion requirements: a meta-analysis. J Clin Anesth 2006;18:124.
117. Rashiq S, Finegan BA, Rashiq S, et al. The effect of spinal anesthesia on blood transfusion rate in total joint arthroplasty. Can J Surg 2006;49:391.
118. Stevens RD, Van Gessel E, Flory N, et al. Lumbar plexus block reduces pain and blood loss associated with total hip arthroplasty. Anesthesiology 2000; 93:115.
119. Chelly JE, Greger J, Gebhard R, et al. Continuous femoral blocks improve recovery and outcome of patients undergoing total knee arthroplasty. J Arthroplasty 2001;16:436.
121. Goodnough LT, Brecher ME, Kanter MH, et al. Transfusion medicine. First of two parts–blood transfusion. N Engl J Med 1999;340:438.
120. Goodnough LT, Brecher ME, Kanter MH, et al. Transfusion medicine. Second of two parts–blood conservation. N Engl J Med 1999;340:525.
122. Shander A, Hofmann A, Ozawa S, et al. Activity-based costs of blood transfusions in surgical patients at four hospitals. Transfusion 2010;50:753.
123. Callesen T, Bech K, Kehlet H, et al. Prospective study of chronic pain after groin hernia repair. Br J Surg 1999;86:1528.
124. Borly L, Anderson IB, Bardram L, et al. Preoperative prediction model of outcome after cholecystectomy for symptomatic gallstones. Scand J Gastroenterol 1999;34:1144.
125. Tasmuth T, Kataja M, Blomqvist C, et al. Treatment-related factors predisposing to chronic pain in patients with breast cancer–a multivariate approach. Acta Oncol 1997;36:625.
126. Katz J, Jackson M, Kavanagh BP, et al. Acute pain after thoracic surgery predicts long-term post-thoracotomy pain. Clin J Pain 1996;12:50.
127. Kalso E, Perttunen K, Kaasinen S, et al. Pain after thoracic surgery. Acta Anaesthesiol Scand 1992;36:96.
128. Bates T, Ebbs SR, Harrison M, et al. Influence of cholecystectomy on symptoms. Br J Surg 1991;78:964.
129. Kroner K, Krebs B, Skov J, et al. Immediate and long-term phantom breast syndrome after mastectomy: incidence, clinical characteristics and relationship to pre-mastectomy breast pain. Pain 1989;36:327.
130. Bach S, Noreng MF, Tjellden NU, et al. Phantom limb pain in amputees during the first 12 months following limb amputation, after preoperative lumbar epidural blockade. Pain 1988;33:297.
131. Perkins FM, Kehlet H, Perkins FM, et al. Chronic pain as an outcome of surgery. A review of predictive factors. Anesthesiology 2000;93:1123.

132. Obata H, Saito S, Fujita N, et al. Epidural block with mepivacaine before surgery reduces long-term post-thoracotomy pain. Can J Anaesth 1999;46:1127.

133. Stephens J, Laskin B, Pashos C, et al. The burden of acute postoperative pain and the potential role of the COX-2-specific inhibitors. Rheumatology 2003; 42(Suppl 3):iii40.

134. Stewart WF, Ricci JA, Chee E, et al. Lost productive time and cost due to common pain conditions in the US workforce. JAMA 2003;290:2443.

Local Anesthetic Systemic Toxicity: Prevention and Treatment

Pilar Mercado, MD[a],*, Guy L. Weinberg, MD[a,b]

KEYWORDS

- Local anesthetic • Toxicity • Treatment • Prevention
- Intralipid • Lipid emulsion

Anesthesia is a sine qua non for most surgeries. From the earliest days of anesthesia practice and the first use of regional anesthesia, this specialty has aimed to alleviate pain, make surgery tolerable, and thereby allow advances in operative technique and extend the curative reach of surgical practice. In the 130 years since the introduction of regional anesthesia, the bar has been pushed from simply producing brief surgical anesthesia to providing long-lasting pain control, even sending patients home with continuous local anesthetic (LA) infusions to control postoperative pain for days.

Like any medical advance, progress in regional anesthesia has not come without its share of complications, including a spectrum extending from localized nerve injury to systemic cardiovascular (CV) toxicity and death. Isolated in 1859 and first used as a topical anesthetic for ocular surgery by Carl Koller in 1884, cocaine rapidly gained widespread favor. However, the systemic toxic effects of cocaine were quickly identified and became the subject of an insightful review before the Kings County Medical Society by Mattison in 1887. The investigator cautioned that cocaine's "potency for good implies a potency for harm."[1]

Although the clinical picture of LA systemic toxicity (LAST) takes many forms, the earliest descriptions of its main features as involving respiratory failure and seizures along with "palpitations and irregular heart action"[1] can hardly be improved. Cocaine's toxicity was the impetus for the development of safer synthetic LAs. However, the development of these LAs did not eliminate LAST entirely, and when bupivacaine and etidocaine, 2 highly lipophilic drugs, were later introduced into clinical practice,

---

The authors have nothing to disclose.

[a] Department of Anesthesiology, University of Illinois at Chicago, 3200 West UICH MC 515, 1740 West Taylor Street, Chicago, IL 60612, USA
[b] Department of Anesthesiology, Jesse Brown Veterans Affairs Medical Center, 820 South Damen Avenue, Bed Tower Room 2677, Chicago, IL 60612, USA
* Corresponding author.
E-mail address: Pmerca1@uic.edu

Anesthesiology Clin 29 (2011) 233–242
doi:10.1016/j.anclin.2011.04.007
1932-2275/11/$ – see front matter © 2011 Elsevier Inc. All rights reserved.
anesthesiology.theclinics.com

there was a resurgence in the awareness of serious complications related to regional anesthesia with these drugs.

Since Albright's seminal editorial calling attention to the problem, substantial basic laboratory research, including in vitro and intact animal studies, has focused on possible mechanisms of systemic toxicity as well as potential treatments. Practical, statistical, and ethical considerations preclude meaningful randomized controlled clinical trials. Nevertheless, benchwork has focused for more than 30 years on several relevant issues, such as the development of less toxic but effective LAs, understanding the mechanisms of LA toxicity, development of vehicles for safer delivery of LA to the site of action, prevention of LAST, and, more recently, treatment of LAST, particularly with intravenous (IV) lipid emulsion (LE).

LAST
Mechanisms and Clinical Presentation

Hypoxia and acidosis have been documented to exacerbate cardiac toxicity of LAs,[2,3] possibly as a result of LA ion trapping, worsened oxidative phosphorylation in oxygen-deprived tissues, or both. In his 1979 report of a healthy young man who suffered cardiac arrest after caudal anesthesia with etidocaine, Prentiss[4] suggested that the drug's lipophilicity and large capacity for protein binding could account for persistence in the myocardium and direct myocardial toxicity as evidenced by resistance to countershock during resuscitation. Later that year, Albright's[5] editorial reviewing cardiac arrest seen with etidocaine and bupivacaine focused on the almost-simultaneous manifestation of central nervous system (CNS) and cardiac toxicities seen with these agents, emphasizing that hypoxia alone could not have been a causative factor. This finding launched the major interest in debate and research on LAST that continues to the present.

It is clear from Butterworth's[6] extensive review of mechanisms of LA cardiac toxicity that the underlying mechanism of this toxicity remains elusive. A discussion of the myriad possibilities is beyond the scope of this article, and the reader is referred to the investigator's review. LAs are classically viewed as exerting clinically relevant effects because of their binding and inhibition of voltage-gated sodium channels. What happens then, however, can vary because the channels come in multiple distinct forms and undergo differential conformational change depending on the drug that binds it.[7] LAs also affect a variety of other ionotropic and metabotropic signaling systems, as well as mitochondrial metabolism and oxidative phosphorylation. Weinberg and colleagues[8] demonstrated that bupivacaine inhibits the mitochondrial enzyme carnitine-acylcarnitine translocase, effectively preventing state III respiration and the cardiac myocyte's use of fatty acids as fuel. These diverse adverse cellular effects are now thought to contribute to the many signs and symptoms of LAST. The effects at target sites are somewhat stereospecific, and the single enantiomer preparations levobupivacaine and ropivacaine are considered less toxic. However, the clinical relevance of these preparations' presumed differential toxicity and safety is arguable because severe LAST has been described with both drugs.[9,10]

The initial clinical presentation of LAST varies widely, sometimes occurring without the classic premonitory signs and symptoms expected, such as tinnitus, perioral tingling, or slurred speech.[11] Factors influencing the clinical picture of LAST are complex, and the resulting symptoms are unpredictable, depending on the interaction of patient factors (comorbidities), the specifics of LA administration (site of injection, dose, volume, and so forth), and the particular LA used. The more potent anesthetics, such as bupivacaine and etidocaine, are more likely to cause lethal arrhythmias than the less potent lidocaine, whereas lidocaine may cause CV toxicity via depressed contractility.[12–14] In other words, the clinical picture of systemic toxicity may take different forms depending on which LA is used.[6] Notably, anesthetic potency and toxicity are both tightly linked to the lipophilicity of LA. The doses required to achieve both CNS and cardiac toxicities tend to be similar with the more potent lipophilic drugs.

It is widely recognized that the heart and CNS differ with respect to their relative thresholds for toxicity. The heart is classically viewed as being more intrinsically resistant to the toxic effects of LAs than the CNS, explaining why manifestations of CNS toxicity are usually seen first in the LAST syndrome. Differential sensitivity could be because of greater density of potential targets or a greater requirement for aerobic metabolism in the brain. Alternatively, classic pharmacokinetic/dynamic explanation could hold that delivery of LA to CNS targets could supercede or precede that in the heart. CNS effects include signs and symptoms of excitation, which include prodromes of dizziness, tinnitus, circumoral numbness, muscle twitching, and slurred speech, leading to frank seizures. CNS depression can also occur, presenting with respiratory depression, obtundation, and coma. This depression is thought to be because of neuronal desynchronization secondary to disturbances in γ-aminobutyric acid neurotransmission.[15] Cardiac toxicity is similarly described as occurring in 2 phases. Initially, central activation of the sympathetic nervous system results in hypertension and tachycardia, potentially masking the direct cardiodepressant effects of LA. Eventually, depressed contractility leads to progressive hypotension. In addition, arrhythmias are common and typically malignant, persistent, and resistant to standard treatment. Arrhythmias can include both tachyarrhythmia and severe brady-dysrhythmia that can progress to frank CV collapse.[16]

Prevention

Prevention of unintended adverse consequences is the crux of improving patient safety during regional anesthesia or any procedure for that matter. Practices such as incremental injection, frequent aspiration, use of a tracer, and, possibly, ultrasound guidance can improve safety. Systemic toxicity results from increased plasma concentration of LA above a threshold level, usually from either direct intravascular injection or after systemic absorption of drug from a tissue depot. Therefore, the detection of needle or catheter placement in a blood vessel is of paramount importance before injecting potentially toxic doses of LA. Furthermore, it is important to understand that greater caution should be exercised in patients with cardiac disease, renal impairment, or metabolic disease, which likely reduces the threshold for LAST. Notably, many of these ideas are not new.[17]

Practice standards for regional anesthesia are intended to reduce the risk of LA toxicity.[18] These practices include limiting the dose of LA to the smallest volume and concentration necessary to achieve blockade; fractionated injection and frequent aspiration to detect intravascular placement of the needle; use of a marker of intravascular injection, such as epinephrine or fentanyl[19,20]; and continual communication with the patient to detect early signs and symptoms of intravascular or intraneural injection. It is equally important to proceed with more caution in those patients deemed to be at higher risk because patients with conduction abnormalities, low cardiac output or ischemia, metabolic disease, liver disease, low plasma protein concentration, and acidosis (increased free fraction of LA) are likely to have lower thresholds for toxicity.

Although sound practice, these guidelines alone cannot prevent all occurrences of LAST. A high index of suspicion is necessary to detect IV injection before toxicity is apparent. Although negative aspiration may detect most intravascular injections (particularly in multiorifice catheters),[21] it can prove false with single-orifice catheters[22] or in peripheral nerve blockade[23,24] in general. The addition of epinephrine, 5 μg/mL, serves as an effective marker of IV injection, causing increase in heart rate.[19] However, the classic epinephrine test dose is not without controversy, and false-positives during labor epidural placement may lead to unnecessary removal of a correctly placed catheter as well as further attempts at placement.[21] The test dose with epinephrine is also unreliable in the elderly or in patients taking β-blockers, although an increase in systolic blood pressure can still be seen.[19] Fentanyl is a reliable marker in laboring women, and 100 μg of the drug administered intravenously causes drowsiness, sedation, or dizziness with a sensitivity and positive predictive value of greater than 80%.[20]

From experience, it is known that there is likely a subgroup of patients in whom even doses considered normally safe can be harmful.[25] The advent of ultrasound guidance may allow greater precision during peripheral nerve blockade and deposition of smaller volumes of LA.[26] Although in this scenario less is more, ultrasound-guided regional anesthesia (USGRA) has not eliminated risk of LAST,[18] and one should remain cognizant of the potential for misleading visual artifacts during ultrasonography.[27] However, USGRA can help the operator detect intravascular or intraneural injection in real-time, thus potentially limiting harm.[24,28,29]

Treatment

Severe LAST is a rare event. The rarity of this condition precludes meaningful prospective study in humans, and until the last few years, treatment of CV collapse was solely supportive, with standard advanced cardiac life support/basic life support (ACLS/BLS) and cardiopulmonary bypass for patients resistant to resuscitation. Prompt recognition of LAST, preferably early in the toxic syndrome, can prevent further progression if injection is halted and allow the clinician to prepare for what may follow. It has been recognized for some time that although hypoxemia and acidosis in this setting do not necessarily cause CV toxicity, per se, they can certainly worsen the outcome.[2,30] Therefore, maintenance of oxygenation and effective cardiopulmonary resuscitation (CPR) to conserve organ perfusion until plasma levels of LA decrease remains a cornerstone of treatment. Benzodiazepines or a small dose of propofol can be given to raise the seizure threshold if seizures occur, although the use of propofol is not recommended in cases of hemodynamic compromise.

LE therapy (LET) is now solidly part of the algorithm to treat LAST (the American Society of Regional Anesthesia and Pain Medicine Practice Advisory) (**Box 1**). Initially proposed as a final effort in resuscitation after failed conventional therapy,[31] the efficacy of LET after early or immediate use to prevent progression of toxicity has been described in multiple case reports.[32–38] The essential elements of LET are administration of a bolus, which can be repeated after 5 minutes for 2 or more times for persistent circulatory collapse, followed by continuous infusion for at least 10 minutes after return of CV stability.[18] The infusion is crucial[39] because recurrence of systemic toxicity after successful treatment with LET has been described.[40] Marwick and colleagues[40] reported a case of recurrence of CV instability 40 minutes after completion of the Intralipid (Fresenius Kabi, AG, Bad Homburg, Germany) infusion, complicated by the unavailability of additional LE. This case underscores the importance of having sufficient amounts of LE, as much as 1000 mL, readily available. Close observation for signs of hemodynamic compromise for at least 12 hours is recommended to anticipate that further treatment with lipid could be required.

Standard resuscitation measures include the use of vasopressors. However, there is evidence from rodent studies that standard or repeated doses of epinephrine or vasopressin may impair resuscitation with lipid and result in worse metabolic profiles.[41–43]

Box 1
Practice advisory on treatment of LAST

For patients experiencing signs or symptoms of LAST

- Get help
- Initial focus
  - Airway management: ventilate with 100% oxygen
  - Seizure suppression: benzodiazepines are preferred
  - BLS/ACLS may require prolonged effort
- Infuse 20% LE (values in parenthesis are for a 70-kg patient)
  - Bolus 1.5 mL/kg (lean body mass) intravenously longer than 1 minute (approximately 100 mL)
  - Continuous infusion at 0.25 mL/kg/min (approximately 18 mL/min; adjust by roller clamp)
  - Repeat bolus once or twice for persistent CV collapse
  - Double the infusion rate to 0.5 mL/kg/min if blood pressure remains low
  - Continue infusion for at least 10 minutes after attaining circulatory stability
  - Recommended upper limit: approximately 10 mL/kg LE over the first 30 minutes
- Avoid vasopressin, calcium channel blockers, β-blockers, or LA
- Alert the nearest facility having cardiopulmonary bypass capability
- Avoid propofol in patients having signs of CV instability
- Post LAST events at www.lipidrescue.org and report use of lipid to www.lipidregistry.org

---

Epinephrine given in smaller than usual doses (<5 µg/kg) proved beneficial in an animal model of bupivacaine cardiac toxicity, whereas LE alone was also more effective than epinephrine or vasopressin alone or in combination in a rodent model of LAST.[42] Conflicting studies exist that demonstrate worse outcomes with LET in the presence of vasopressor use in a porcine model.[44,45] Confounding results may stem from the particular model in which the drugs used to induce anesthesia in swine may cause hemodynamic and electrophysiologic effects not seen in the rodent model.[46]

In the specific setting of asphyxial (not LA- induced) cardiac arrest in rabbits, LE actually impaired return of spontaneous circulation.[47] Hypoxia was also a component and, therefore, a confounding element in the study by Mayr and colleagues[44] comparing epinephrine and vasopressin with LET. Animal models of lipid rescue for LA toxicity assume adequate oxygenation, as is the case in the multiple reports of successful use in humans.[9,48–50] In the setting of LAST, it is expected that airway management begins at the first sign of toxicity, and use of LET similarly begins when the patient is well oxygenated and ventilated (and receiving effective CPR if necessary). It is important to note that a decrease in pH lowers the affinity of bupivacaine and ropivacaine for LE.[51]

Adverse Effects of LE

With any treatment physicians must ask themselves, "What is the potential harm to the patient? Am I making things worse?" The general sense of clinical experience at this point suggests that any potential risk from the use of LE is far outweighed by its benefit in preventing the prospect of CV collapse, which is often refractory to conventional treatment. Published reports of complications after use of LE given as parenteral nutrition focus on allergy, hyperthermia, pancreatitis, hypercoagulability, antineutro-phil activity, and elevated liver enzyme levels,[52,53] as well as fat embolism in infants.[54] At present, there are no reports in the literature of clinically significant complications resulting from LET. Hyperamylasemia was reported in a person treated with lipid for LA toxicity, although it did not progress to clinical pancreatitis.[40] There are 2 published reports of LET in children with LAST-associated cardiotoxicity: one in a 13-year-old adolescent and one in a 40-day-old term infant.[49,55] Both cases resulted in a return of normal hemodynamics without apparent adverse effects of the lipid infusion. None-theless, medical experience with this intervention is still in the early phase, and the overall safety profile of LET remains to be seen. The recent discovery that the median lethal dose of high-volume LE in rats is an order of magnitude higher than the doses used in humans[56] is encouraging.

Despite the efficacy of this antidote to LAST, it is not know with certainty how it works. Weinberg and colleagues[57] postulated that LE might act as a lipid sink, pulling lipophilic drugs out of susceptible tissues. There is also evidence from an isolated rat heart model that lipid infusion may have a direct positive inotropic effect on the myocardium,[58] which may be because of the activation of calcium channels in cardiac myocytes.[59] Improvement or restoration of metabolism may also play a role in the beneficial effect of LE, as suggested by work in animal models of myocardial ischemia[60,61] and reversal of bupivacaine's inhibition of mitochondrial fatty acid trans-port at concentrations too low to provide a sink.[62]

Not all formulations of LE are identical, and their relative efficacies in treating LAST and potential for causing side effects are not known. Intralipid is the most commonly reported emulsion in animal studies and case reports. Intralipid is a soy-based LE con-taining mostly long-chain triglycerides (LCTs). There is evidence that LCT emulsions more effectively bind long-acting LAs than mixed LCT/medium-chain triglyceride (MCT) emulsions.[51] However, LCT/MCT formulations have also been used to treat LAST effectively in humans and without deleterious consequences; Liposyn (Hospira, Lake Forest, IL, USA) and Medialipid (B. Braun, Melsungen, Germany) are 2 such emul-sions. Candela and colleagues[63] recently demonstrated the efficacy of both LCT and LCT/MCT emulsions in piglets with bupivacaine-induced cardiac electrophysiologic changes, but in this case, the emulsions were compared with saline alone, not to each other. Further investigation is warranted to allow the tailoring of LET more precisely.

FUTURE TRENDS

The search to develop safe, effective, long-lasting pain control with minimal side effects has led to the development of controlled-release vehicles for the delivery of LA to its site of action. Two such promising carriers are liposomes and microparticles. Liposomes are lipid bilayers with aqueous centers, whereas microparticles are composed of biodegradable polymers.[64] Encapsulation of LA by these vehicles allows slower release into surrounding tissue, prolonging duration of action and reducing peak plasma concentrations of LA, potentially decreasing risk of systemic cardiac and neurotoxicity.[65,66] Mimicking an accidental intravascular injection, Boogaerts and colleagues[67] compared systemic toxicity of liposome-encapsulated bupivacaine to bupivacaine with and without epinephrine injected into rabbits. The threshold for the appearance of signs of toxicity was significantly higher in the liposome group. Tofoli and colleagues[65] demonstrated that liposome-encapsulated mepivacaine has a longer half-life than either plain or epinephrine-associated LA when injected into the oral mucosa of rats. Local tissue inflammation was also less in the liposome group 4 days after injection, suggesting a protective effect.

In addition to a potentially better safety profile, encapsulation also allows the use of compounds that have anesthetic properties other than traditional LA but that might otherwise be too potent, or toxic, to use on their own.[66] Tetrodotoxin and saxitoxin (STX) are site 1 sodium-channel blockers that must be used in very small doses to avoid systemic toxicity. Used in liposomes, STX resulted in sciatic nerve block lasting for days without significant systemic or local toxicity, whereas myotoxicity was seen in formulations containing bupivacaine.[66]

Although research to date has involved mainly in vitro and in vivo animal studies, preliminary work in humans is promising. Liposome-encapsulated bupivacaine injected into the epidural space of a patient with cancer resulted in extended pain relief without hemodynamic compromise or motor blockade.[68] Of course, potential problems exist with these delivery systems. Apart from being neurotoxic, LAs are known to be myotoxic as well. The incorporation of bupivacaine into microparticles caused a greater degree of myotoxicity when injected into the sciatic nerves of rats compared with bupivacaine alone,[69] which may be because of an indirect effect of the microparticle. Specifically, LA deposited as part of such a formulation tends to stay at the site of action longer, and prolonged exposure to bupivacaine, even at lower plasma concentrations or low release rates from the vehicle, can result in local toxicity. Another concern with such formulations is potential leakage of large doses of LA from the vehicle instead of slow release. However, liposomal preparations can be precisely tailored by changing lipid composition, changing size,[64] or the addition of other drugs that affect LA release, such as dexamethasone.[66] Continued progress toward developing better safer LA delivery systems will broaden the practice of regional anesthesia and add an important dimension to its many applications.

REFERENCES

1. American Association for the Advancement of Science, Highwire Press. In: Science, vol. 9. New York: Moses King; 1887. p. 329.
2. Moore DC, Crawford RD, Scurlock JE. Severe hypoxia and acidosis following local anesthetic-induced convulsions. Anesthesiology 1980;53(3):259–60.
3. Moore DC, Thompson GE, Crawford RD. Long-acting local anesthetic drugs and convulsions with hypoxia and acidosis. Anesthesiology 1982;56(3):230–2.
4. Prentiss JE. Cardiac arrest following caudal anesthesia. Anesthesiology 1979; 50(1):51–3.
5. Albright GA. Cardiac arrest following regional anesthesia with etidocaine or bupivacaine. Anesthesiology 1979;51(4):285–7.
6. Butterworth JF. Models and mechanisms of local anesthetic cardiac toxicity: a review. Reg Anesth Pain Med 2010;35(2):167–76.
7. Fukuda K, Nakajima T, Viswanathan PC, et al. Compound-specific Na+ channel pore conformational changes induced by local anaesthetics. J Physiol 2005; 564(Pt 1):21–31.
8. Weinberg GL, Palmer JW, VadeBoncouer TR, et al. Bupivacaine inhibits acylcarnitine exchange in cardiac mitochondria. Anesthesiology 2000;92(2): 523–8.
9. Litz RJ, Popp M, Stehr SN, et al. Successful resuscitation of a patient with ropivacaine-induced asystole after axillary plexus block using lipid infusion. Anaesthesia 2006;61:800–1.
10. Foxall G, McCahon R, Lamb J, et al. Levobupivacaine-induced seizures and cardiovascular collapse treated with Intralipid. Anaesthesia 2007;62(5): 516–8.

11. Di Gregorio G, Neal JM, Rosenquist RW, et al. Clinical presentation of local anesthetic systemic toxicity: a review of published cases, 1979 to 2009. Reg Anesth Pain Med 2010;35(2):181–7.
12. de Jong RH, Ronfeld RA, DeRosa RA. Cardiovascular effects of convulsant and supraconvulsant doses of amide local anesthetics. Anesth Analg 1982;61(1): 3–9.
13. Chadwick HS. Toxicity and resuscitation in lidocaine- or bupivacaine-infused cats. Anesthesiology 1985;63(4):385–90.
14. Feldman HS, Arthur GR, Covino BG. Comparative systemic toxicity of convulsant and supraconvulsant doses of intravenous ropivacaine, bupivacaine, and lidocaine in the conscious dog. Anesth Analg 1989;69(6):794–801.
15. Veering BT. Complications and local anaesthetic toxicity in regional anaesthesia. Curr Opin Anaesthesiol 2003;16(5):455–9.
16. Adverse reactions with bupivacaine. FDA Drug Bull 1983;13(3):23.
17. Drasner K. Local anesthetic systemic toxicity: a historical perspective. Reg Anesth Pain Med 2010;35(2):162–6.
18. Neal JM, Bernards CM, Butterworth JF, et al. ASRA practice advisory on local anesthetic systemic toxicity. Reg Anesth Pain Med 2010;35(2):152–61.
19. Moore DC, Batra MS. The components of an effective test dose prior to epidural block. Anesthesiology 1981;55(6):693–6.
20. Guay J. The epidural test dose: a review. Anesth Analg 2006;102(3):921–9.
21. Norris MC, Ferrenbach D, Dalman H, et al. Does epinephrine improve the diagnostic accuracy of aspiration during labor epidural analgesia? Anesth Analg 1999;88(5): 1073–6.
22. Kenepp NB, Gutsche BB. Inadvertent intravascular injections during lumbar epidural anesthesia. Anesthesiology 1981;54(2):172–3.
23. Zetlaoui PJ, Labbe JP, Benhamou D. Ultrasound guidance for axillary plexus block does not prevent intravascular injection. Anesthesiology 2008;108(4):761.
24. VadeBoncouer TR, Weinberg GL, Oswald S, et al. Early detection of intravascular injection during ultrasound-guided supraclavicular brachial plexus block. Reg Anesth Pain Med 2008;33(3):278–9.
25. Weinberg GL, Laurito CE, Geldner P, et al. Malignant ventricular dysrhythmias in a patient with isovaleric acidemia receiving general and local anesthesia for suction lipectomy. J Clin Anesth 1997;9(8):668–70.
26. Eichenberger U, Stockli S, Marhofer P, et al. Minimal local anesthetic volume for peripheral nerve block: a new ultrasound-guided, nerve dimension-based method. Reg Anesth Pain Med 2009;34(3):242–6.
27. Saranteas T, Matsota P, Stachtos G, et al. Duplication of the brachial plexus: an ultrasound refraction artifact? Reg Anesth Pain Med 2010;35(4):405–6.
28. Neal JM, Wedel DJ. Ultrasound guidance and peripheral nerve injury: is our vision as sharp as we think it is? Reg Anesth Pain Med 2010;35(4):335–7.
29. Robards C, Clendenen S, Greengrass R. Intravascular injection during ultrasound-guided axillary block: negative aspiration can be misleading. Anesth Analg 2008;107(5):1754–5.
30. Heavner JE, Dryden CF Jr, Sanghani V, et al. Severe hypoxia enhances central nervous system and cardiovascular toxicity of bupivacaine in lightly anesthetized pigs. Anesthesiology 1992;77(1):142–7.
31. Weinberg G. Lipid infusion resuscitation for local anesthetic toxicity: proof of clinical efficacy. Anesthesiology 2006;105(1):7–8.
32. Markowitz S, Neal JM. Immediate lipid emulsion therapy in the successful treatment of bupivacaine systemic toxicity. Reg Anesth Pain Med 2009;34(3):276.

33. Charbonneau H, Marcou TA, Mazoit J-X, et al. Early use of lipid emulsion to treat incipient mepivacaine intoxication. Reg Anesth Pain Med 2009;34(3):277–8.
34. Sonsino DH, Fischler M. Immediate intravenous lipid infusion in the successful resuscitation of ropivacaine-induced cardiac arrest after infraclavicular brachial plexus block. Reg Anesth Pain Med 2009;34(3):276–7.
35. McCutchen T, Gerancher JC. Early intralipid therapy may have prevented bupivacaine-associated cardiac arrest. Reg Anesth Pain Med 2008;33(2):178–80.
36. Cordell CL, Schubkegel T, Light TR, et al. Lipid infusion rescue for bupivacaine-induced cardiac arrest after axillary block. J Hand Surg Am 2010;35(1):144–6.
37. Espinet AJ, Emmerton MT. The successful use of intralipid for treatment of local anesthetic-induced central nervous system toxicity: some considerations for administration of intralipid in an emergency. Clin J Pain 2009;25(9):808–9.
38. Spence AG. Lipid reversal of central nervous system symptoms of bupivacaine toxicity. Anesthesiology 2007;107(3):516–7.
39. Weinberg GL. Limits to lipid in the literature and lab: what we know, what we don't know. Anesth Analg 2009;108(4):1062–4.
40. Marwick PC, Levin AI, Coetzee AR. Recurrence of cardiotoxicity after lipid rescue from bupivacaine-induced cardiac arrest. Anesth Analg 2009;108(4):1344–6.
41. Weinberg GL, Di Gregorio G, Ripper R, et al. Resuscitation with lipid versus epinephrine in a rat model of bupivacaine overdose. Anesthesiology 2008;108(5):907–13.
42. Di Gregorio G, Schwartz D, Ripper R, et al. Lipid emulsion is superior to vasopressin in a rodent model of resuscitation from toxin-induced cardiac arrest. Crit Care Med 2009;37(3):993–9.
43. Hiller DB, Gregorio GD, Ripper R, et al. Epinephrine impairs lipid resuscitation from bupivacaine overdose: a threshold effect. Anesthesiology 2009;111(3):498–505.
44. Mayr VD, Mitterschiffthaler L, Neurauter A, et al. A comparison of the combination of epinephrine and vasopressin with lipid emulsion in a porcine model of asphyxial cardiac arrest after intravenous injection of bupivacaine. Anesth Analg 2008;106(5):1566–71, Table of contents.
45. Hicks SD, Salcido DD, Logue ES, et al. Lipid emulsion combined with epinephrine and vasopressin does not improve survival in a swine model of bupivacaine-induced cardiac arrest. Anesthesiology 2009;111(1):138–46.
46. Woehlck HJ, El-Orbany M. Anesthetic effects and lipid resuscitation protocols. Anesthesiology 2010;112(2):499–500 [author reply: 500].
47. Harvey M, Cave G, Kazemi A. Intralipid infusion diminishes return of spontaneous circulation after hypoxic cardiac arrest in rabbits. Anesth Analg 2009;108(4):1163–8.
48. Rosenblatt MA, Abel M, Fischer GW, et al. Successful use of a 20% lipid emulsion to resuscitate a patient after a presumed bupivacaine-related cardiac arrest. Anesthesiology 2006;105(1):217–8.
49. Ludot H, Tharin JY, Belouadah M, et al. Successful resuscitation after ropivacaine and lidocaine-induced ventricular arrhythmia following posterior lumbar plexus block in a child. Anesth Analg 2008;106(5):1572–4.
50. Warren J, Brian T, Georgescu A, et al. Intravenous lipid infusion in the successful resuscitation of local anesthetic-induced cardiovascular collapse following supraclavicular brachial plexus block. Anesth Analg 2008;106(5):1578–80.
51. Mazoit JX, Le Guen R, Beloeil H, et al. Binding of long-lasting local anesthetics to lipid emulsions. Anesthesiology 2009;110(2):380–6.
52. Cave G, Harvey M. Intravenous lipid emulsion as antidote beyond local anesthetic toxicity: a systematic review. Acad Emerg Med 2009;16(9):815–24.

53. Driscoll DF. Lipid injectable emulsions: pharmacopeial and safety issues. Pharm Res 2006;23(9):1959–69.
54. Barson AJ, Chistwick ML, Doig CM. Fat embolism in infancy after intravenous fat infusions. Arch Dis Child 1978;53(3):218–23.
55. Shah S, Gopalakrishnan S, Apuya J, et al. Use of Intralipid in an infant with impending cardiovascular collapse due to local anesthetic toxicity. J Anesth 2009;23(3):439–41.
56. Hiller DB, Di Gregorio G, Kelly K, et al. Safety of high volume lipid emulsion infusion: a first approximation of LD50 in rats. Reg Anesth Pain Med 2010; 35(2):140–4.
57. Weinberg GL, Ripper R, Murphy P, et al. Lipid infusion accelerates removal of bupivacaine and recovery from bupivacaine toxicity in the isolated rat heart. Reg Anesth Pain Med 2006;31(4):296–303.
58. Stehr SN, Ziegeler JC, Pexa A, et al. The effects of lipid infusion on myocardial function and bioenergetics in l-bupivacaine toxicity in the isolated rat heart. Anesth Analg 2007;104(1):186–92.
59. Huang JM, Xian H, Bacaner M. Long-chain fatty acids activate calcium channels in ventricular myocytes. Proc Natl Acad Sci U S A 1992;89(14):6452–6.
60. Van de Velde M, Wouters PF, Rolf N, et al. Long-chain triglycerides improve recovery from myocardial stunning in conscious dogs. Cardiovasc Res 1996; 32(6):1008–15.
61. Van de Velde M, DeWolff M, Leather HA, et al. Effects of lipids on the functional and metabolic recovery from global myocardial stunning in isolated rabbit hearts. Cardiovasc Res 2000;48(1):129–37.
62. Stehr SN, Ziegler J, Pexa A, et al. Lipid effects on myocardial function in L-bupivacaine induced toxicity in the isolated rat heart [abstract]. Reg Anesth Pain Med 2005;30:5.
63. Candela D, Louart G, Bousquet P-J, et al. Reversal of bupivacaine-induced cardiac electrophysiologic changes by two lipid emulsions in anesthetized and mechanically ventilated piglets. Anesth Analg 2010;110(5):1473–9.
64. Grant GJ, Bansinath M. Liposomal delivery systems for local anesthetics. Reg Anesth Pain Med 2001;26(1):61–3.
65. Tofoli GR, Cereda CM, de Araujo DR, et al. Pharmacokinetic and local toxicity studies of liposome-encapsulated and plain mepivacaine solutions in rats. Drug Deliv 2010;17(2):68–76.
66. Epstein-Barash H, Shichor I, Kwon AH, et al. Prolonged duration local anesthesia with minimal toxicity. Proc Natl Acad Sci U S A 2009;106(17):7125–30.
67. Boogaerts J, Declercq A, Lafont N, et al. Toxicity of bupivacaine encapsulated into liposomes and injected intravenously: comparison with plain solutions. Anesth Analg 1993;76(3):553–5.
68. Lafont ND, Legros FJ, Boogaerts JG. Use of liposome-associated bupivacaine in a cancer pain syndrome. Anaesthesia 1996;51(6):578–9.
69. Padera R, Bellas E, Tse JY, et al. Local myotoxicity from sustained release of bupivacaine from microparticles. Anesthesiology 2008;108(5):921–8.

Assessment and Treatment of Postblock Neurologic Injury

Alain Borgeat, MD*, José Aguirre, MD

KEYWORDS

- Regional anesthesia • Nerve injury • Electromyography
- Nerve conduction studies

The incidence of peripheral nerve injury after regional anesthesia is low. Different factors have been cited to explain this occurrence. Moreover, it is not uncommon for regional anesthesia to be blamed for postoperative neural complications. Electromyography is the standard to assess nerve damage after regional anesthesia. Therefore, it is mandatory for the anesthesiology to have a good understanding of this technique. The aim of this chapter is to provide the ABC of electroneuromyography that any anesthesiologists performing regional anesthesia should know.

PHYSICAL EXAMINATION

The symptoms of nerve injury after regional anesthesia manifest after the block has worn off. This occurs in most cases within 48 hours, but may occasionally be delayed up to 72 hours or more.[1] The symptoms can be minor, ranging from hypohyperesthesia to light intermittent tingling to major complete sensorimotor deficit. Confounding factors such as postoperative pain, immobility, effects of surgery, application of casts, bandaging should be considered as contributing or causative factors. The intensity and duration of symptoms are also dependent on the severity of the injury. Minor symptoms resolve within a few weeks.[1,2] On the other hand, disability secondary to severe nerve damage may last months, even years, and very rarely may be permanent. The occurrence of painful neuropathic pain is usual after axonotmesis and neurotmesis. The occurrence of early or late complex regional pain syndrome (CRPS) type II is possible. Symptoms of nerve injury may be acute and may not become clinically apparent for a few weeks.[2] The delayed appearance of nerve injury is most often

Financial Support was provided solely from departmental sources.
The investigators have nothing to disclose.
Department of Anesthesiology, Balgrist University Hospital, Forchstrasse 340, 8008 Zurich, Switzerland
* Corresponding author.
E-mail address: alain.borgeat@balgrist.ch

Anesthesiology Clin 29 (2011) 243–256
doi:10.1016/j.anclin.2011.04.004

encountered in the case of local neuroinflammation caused by either the local anesthetic or some bleeding in the vicinity of the nerve. Whatever the cause of the damage, diagnostic workup should follow logical and organized sequences (**Fig. 1**).

Physical examination should include a comprehensive assessment of sensorimotor function. The help of a neurologist is advisable. The possibility of a nerve compression (hematoma) should be excluded early in the workup. Ultrasonography of the suspected area is the first examination of choice. Magnetic resonance imaging (MRI) may be indicated in some cases. The possibility of a vascular injury should be kept in mind and assessment of both arterial (ischemia) and venous (thrombosis) circulation should be performed. If a sudomotor test is available, this investigation may disclose the occurrence of an early CRPS.

ELECTRONEUROMYOGRAPHY

Electroneuromyography is the cornerstone of investigations in cases of postblock neurologic injury. Electrodiagnostic studies originated in the nineteenth century, but have been consistently used only within the past 30 to 40 years. This is because the machines became more sophisticated with computerization, and at the same time, easier to use.

The term electrodiagnostic studies encompasses different tests. The most commonly used in the context of postblock neurologic injury are nerve conductions studies (NCSs) and electromyography (EMG). The term electroneuromyography (ENMG) refers to both NCS and EMG because these 2 tests are nearly always performed together.

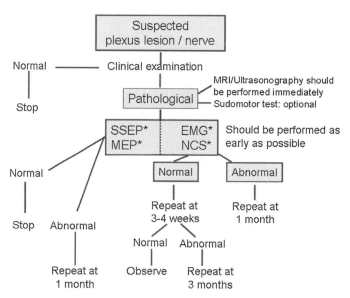

* The choice of the examination will be done according to clinical condition and neuro physiologist's recommendations

Fig. 1. Workup after nerve damage: algorithm. EMG, electromyography; MEP, motor-evoked potential; NCS, nerve conduction study; SSEP, somatosensory-evoked potential. (*From* Borgeat A, Aguirre J, Curt A. Case scenario: neurologic complication after continuous interscalene block. Anesthesiology 2010;112:742–5; with permission.)

NERVE CONDUCTION STUDIES

NCSs record a peripheral neural impulse at some location distant from the site where a propagating action potential is induced in a peripheral nerve. NCS permits assessment of function in motor and sensory nerves. The ability of the nerve to conduct an electrical impulse allows detection of whether a nerve is injured or not. The NCSs most commonly performed are compound muscle action potential (CMAP) for motor nerves, sensory nerve action potential (SNAP) for sensory nerves, compound nerve action potential (CNAP) for mixed (sensory and motor) nerves, and late responses (primary F-waves and H-reflexes).

Understanding of nerve physiology is important when performing NCSs. Nerves conduct impulses through a travelling wave of depolarization along their axon. The axon is the peripheral extension of the proximally located nerve body cell. The cell body is located in the spinal cord for motor cells and peripherally in the dorsal horn ganglion for sensory nerves. While nerves conduct in a physiologic direction (from the spine-motor nerves and to the spine-sensory nerves), if a nerve is electrically stimulated along its course, waves of depolarization travel in both directions. Nerve conduction can be measured orthodromically (physiologic conduction) or antidromically (opposite to the physiologic direction). Usually, NCSs are done only on myelinated nerve fibers because unmyelinated fibers conduct extremely slowly, and therefore, do not contribute significantly to the CMAPs and SNAPs. The myelin plays an important role in nerve conduction. The most important facts to remember about myelin are:

- myelin helps nerves conduct an action potential faster
- the myelin sheath functions as an insulator of the axon
- in myelinated nerves, depolarization occurs only at areas devoid of myelin (nodes of Ranvier); this results in saltatory conduction
- conduction velocity is directly related to internodal length and efficiency of myelin insulation.

Velocities in myelinated nerve range from 40 to 70 m/s. Unmyelinated nerves are much slower, in the range of 1 to 5 m/s. Unmyelinated nerves, in contrast to myelinated nerves, do not conduct through saltatory conduction. They have voltage-dependent sodium channels uniformly throughout the nerves. A demyelinated axon is a myelinated nerve that has lost its myelin covering and therefore it does not become an unmyelinated nerve. This understanding is crucial because although an unmyelinated axon can conduct an impulse along its entire length, a demyelinated axon may not be able to conduct across a demyelinated area. This loss of conduction across a lesion is referred to as conduction block. The term neurapraxia is also used to describe damage where conduction block is present. Following a demyelinating lesion, as part of the recovery phase, there is usually regeneration of immature myelin. It is crucial to emphasize that immature myelin does not insulate as well as mature myelin and therefore, NCSs show a return of conduction but at a slower than normal velocity. Thus, conduction slowing and conduction block indicate demyelination but not axonal damage.

The Action Potential

The action potential is a summation of many potentials. CMAP is the summation of motor units, whereas a SNAP is a summation of individual nerve fibers. Each has its own amplitude and slightly different conduction velocities. The part of the curve that begins to rise first represents the components from the fastest fibers (**Fig. 2**). Other parameters assessed are the amplitude and the duration.

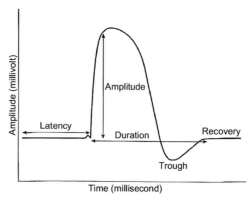

Fig. 2. Normal action potential recording.

Latency

Latency is the time it takes from stimulation of the nerve to the measurement of the beginning of either the SNAP or the CMAP (see **Fig. 2**). The onset latency represents the fastest conducting nerve fibers and the through latency represents the slowest fibers. A latency measurement without a standardized or recorded distance is meaningless.

Conducting velocity

The conducting velocity tells us how fast the nerve is propagating an action potential. It is calculated according to the relation: velocity = distance/time. Motor neurons conduct across a myoneural conduction, therefore the conduction velocity cannot be measured directly, as is the case with sensory neurons, but the following formula should be used: velocity = change in distance/change in time. This implies that at least 2 sites of the same nerve should be stimulated.

Amplitude

The amplitude of CMAP represents the sum of the amplitude of individual potentials. The amplitude is dependent on the integrity of the axon, the muscle fibers it depolarizes, and on the extent of variability of the conduction velocity of individual fibers. Therefore, in the case of a CMAP with low amplitude, it is crucial to distinguish whether this is occurring because of temporal dispersion (variability of the conduction velocity of individual fibers) or is caused by a decreased number of axons. One way to find out whether temporal dispersion or prolongation is the reason is to appreciate the area under the curve. This is an alternative way to estimate the number of axons/muscle fibers that are depolarized.

Duration

The duration is the time from onset latency to termination latency. The duration may be increased in some demyelinating neuropathies with nerve fibers affected differently (temporal dispersion). In general temporal dispersion is observed in acquired as opposed to congenital neuropathies.

Late Responses

H-reflex

The H-reflex is a monosynaptic spinal reflex involving both motor and sensory fibers. This is a sensitive measure to assess radiculopathy. The H-reflex helps to assess proximal lesions, it becomes abnormal relatively early in the development of radiculopathy and finally it incorporates sensory fiber function proximal to the dorsal root ganglion. Clinically H-reflex is very useful to distinguish S1 from L5 radiculopathies, which have similar EMG recordings, but it is also indicated for all radiculopathies.

F-reflex

F-waves are a low-amplitude late response believed to be caused by antidromic motor neurons (anterior horn cells), which then cause an orthodromic impulse to pass back along the motor axons involved. The most widely used parameter is the latency of the shortest reproducible response. However its clinical use has not turned out to be as sensitive as initially hoped.

Clinical Use

NCSs are an important means to evaluate the functional integrity of peripheral nerves (**Box 1**). Abnormal recordings can be seen early (within the first 2–3 days) after a nerve lesion occurs. NCSs enable focal nerve damage to be localized in patients with a mononeuropathy. Localized peripheral nerve damage is characterized by reduced or changed abnormality in amplitude depending on the site of stimulation and recording. Conduction velocity may also be altered (slowing). Combined with EMG, NCSs can determine whether a nerve injury is complete or incomplete and therefore provides information about the prognosis and the likely course of recovery. In the case of a complete lesion, motor units cannot be activated volitionally in a distal muscle. Stimulation of the nerve proximal to the lesion does not elicit a response in muscles supplied by branches arising distal to a complete injury. In the case of a partial lesion, a smaller response can be elicited. However, electrical stimulation distal to the site of, for example, a complete nerve transsection continues to elicit a distal response until wallerian degeneration of the distal nerve stump occurs[3] (generally within 5–10 days). NCSs may discover subclinical polyneuropathy in patients with a mononeuropathy. This is of paramount importance because these patients may be more susceptible to the neurotoxic effects of local anesthetics.[4] Moreover, NCSs may indicate whether the underlying pathologic process is axon loss, characterized by small compound muscle and very little change in conduction velocity, and electromyographically by signs of denervation, or demyelination, characterized by greatly slowed nerve conduction velocity or a conduction block. In this case some or all axons in the nerve become unable to transmit impulses through a segment of nerve but can work more distally. Stimulation proximal to the block leads to a smaller muscle response compared with stimulation performed more distally.

EMG

EMG testing deals with the evaluation of the electrical activity of a muscle and is one of the cornerstones of the electrodiagnostic evaluation of a patient.

Box 1
Nerve conduction studies: clinical information

- Localization of a focal nerve lesion
- Severity of a nerve lesion (complete or incomplete)
- Reveal the presence of an underlying polyneuropathy
- Suggest whether the underlying pathologic process is axon loss or demyelination

Muscle Physiology

EMG assesses skeletal or voluntary muscles. The strength of a contraction is caused by the extrafusal muscle fibers. These fibers are relaxed at rest with an intracellular resting potential of -80 mV. The muscle fiber is surrounded by a plasma membrane, the sarcolemma. The action potential coming from a motor nerve fiber synapses at the neuromuscular junction and then propagates along the sarcolemma. This membrane has extensions into t-tubules, responsible for the release of calcium. The release of calcium, through the actin-myosin system, results in muscle contraction. EMG is the means to measure electrical activation of the muscle fibers.

Motor Units

The motor unit is the fundamental structure that is assessed in electromyography. A motor unit consists of 1 anterior horn cell, its axon, and all the muscle fibers innervated by that motor neuron. The type I motor units refer to those firing first when a person starts to contract a muscle. Those fibers are the smallest. As the contraction increases, there is an orderly recruitment of larger motor units.

EMG Examination

The EMG examination consists of the analysis of 4 components: insertional activity, examination of muscle at rest, analyzing the motor unit, and recruitment.

Insertional activity

Insertional activity deals with the muscle at rest. Healthy muscle at rest is electronically silent as soon as needle movement stops or when the end-plate region is avoided. Normal insertional activity only lasts a few hundred milliseconds, reflecting the needle movement itself. Decreased insertional activity (at the time of needle insertion) is observed in the case of atrophic muscle. Increased insertional activity is suggestive of muscle pathology and is shown by the presence of positive sharp waves and fibrillation potential (**Fig. 3**).

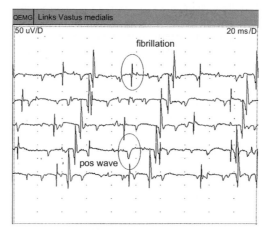

Fig. 3. Abnormal EMG recording showing fibrillation waves und positive waves. (*From* Borgeat A, Aguirre J, Curt A. Case scenario: neurologic complication after continuous interscalene block. Anesthesiology 2010;112:742–5; with permission.)

Examination of the muscle at rest
Normal muscles are electrically silent after needle insertion and the initial short period of insertional activity has vanished.

Spontaneous activity Spontaneous activity is clearly abnormal and occurs in the presence of a pathologic condition. After injury, the membrane potential (resting membrane potential is around −80 mV) becomes more positive because of an increased influx of Na^+ into the damaged cell membrane. Therefore, the muscle cell, being less negative, gets closer to the potential needed for the generation of spontaneous action potentials, which occurs when the cell resting membrane potential is around −60 mV. Examples of abnormal spontaneous potentials are positive sharp waves, fibrillations, complex repetitive discharges, and myotonic discharges. Positive sharp waves (PSWs) are typically muscle fiber action potentials that can be recorded from a muscle with impaired muscle innervation or from an injured portion of a muscle. Fibrillation potentials (FIB) represent the spontaneous action potentials of single muscle fibers firing autonomously in the case of impaired innervation. These abnormal recordings (PSWs and FIBs) most often indicate a process of acute or ongoing impaired innervation. However, these potentials may not be seen on the EMG until 3 weeks or more after an injury.

End-plate region Healthy muscles have no spontaneous activity, as long as the needle avoids the end-plate area. Three types of wave recordings are suggestive of the position of the needle in the end-plate region. These are miniature end-plate potentials (MEPPs), end-plate spikes, and pain. It is important to recognize these features because they can be the source of possible interpretation errors. The end plates should also be avoided because they greatly increase patient discomfort.

Analyzing the motor unit
The analysis of the motor unit follows the assessment of muscle insertional activity and activity at rest. The motor unit includes the following parameters: amplitude, rise time, duration, and phases (**Fig. 4**).

Amplitude In a healthy motor unit, all of the muscle fibers discharge in close synchrony. The greatest contribution in the amplitude in motor unit potential is given by the fibers located close to the tip of the needle. Their contribution decreases as the distance from the needle tip increases. Amplitude of the motor units may be normal, increased, or decreased. Increased amplitude suggests reinnervation (neuropathic

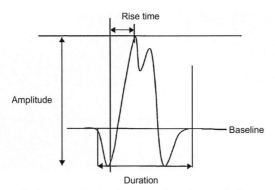

Fig. 4. Motor unit including amplitude, rise time, duration, and phases.

injuries after a few months). On the other hand, myopathies are associated with decreased amplitude.

Rise time This period is the time lag from the peak of the initial positive deflection to the subsequent negative upward peak (see **Fig. 4**). Rise time of about 0.5 milliseconds or less is considered acceptable.

Duration Normal duration is about 5 to 15 milliseconds and is measured from the initial departure from baseline to the initial return to baseline (see **Fig. 4**). This parameter indicates the degree of synchrony of firing among all individual muscle fibers. The duration is short when all the fibers of a motor unit fire in relative synchrony. In the case of asynchrony, as seen in reinnervation, the duration is longer. On the contrary, myopathies are associated with decreased duration because fewer muscle fibers contribute to the motor unit.

Phases A phase is the portion of the waveform between the successive crossings of the baseline. The number of phases equals the number of baseline crossings plus 1. Polyphasic motor units (more than 4 phases) suggest desynchronized discharge or drop-off of individual fibers. According to the needle used, normal muscles have about 10% polyphasic motor unit action potentials (MUAPs) (concentric needle) or 25% polyphasic MUAPs (monopolar needle).

Recruitment
Recruitment refers to the orderly addition of motor units to increase the force of a contraction. There are 2 ways to increase the force of contraction: either by increasing the rate of firing or by mobilizing new units to start firing. To recruit new motor units, motor units, which are normally fired at 5 Hz, are fired at 10 Hz. The recruitment ratio is the rate of firing of the most rapidly firing motor unit (in Hertz) divided by the number of units firing. A recruitment ratio of more than 8 is considered abnormal and suggests a neurogenic process.

Neuropathic recruitment is observed in neuropathies, radiculopathies, motor neuron disease, and nerve trauma (**Fig. 5**). In these situations, the firing rate of these MUAPs is greater than 20 Hz (instead 10 Hz in normal conditions) and may increase to more than 30 Hz. This is explained by the fact that in neuropathic lesions, the number of functional motor units is small (**Fig. 6**). In cases of myopathies, the term early recruitment is used. In this situation, a large number of motor units are recruited to provide a minimal contraction.

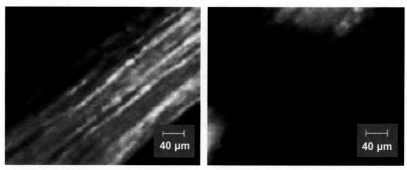

Fig. 5. The saphenous nerve before and after crush. The crush induces a rapid loss of fluorescence at the sight of injury.

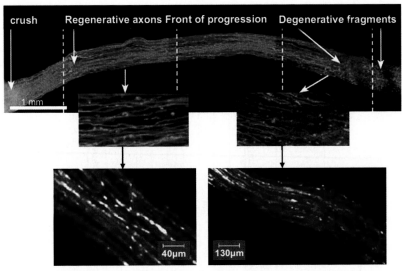

crush   Regenerative axons Front of progression   Degenerative fragments

1 mm

40µm   130µm

Fig. 6. Epifluorescence microscopy of the saphenous nerve 4 days after crush.

Clinical Use

As discussed earlier certain findings are suggestive of denervation. However, abnormal spontaneous activity and increased insertion activity are not pathognomonic of denervation, but may also occur in muscle or neuromuscular function disorders. Moreover, abnormal activity or tracings change during the course of the disease, therefore findings must be related to the temporal profile of (nerve) injury (**Table 1**). Therefore, electromyographic examination is useful for indicating whether weakness has a neurogenic basis and in defining the extent of nerve injury. Electromyographic recordings distinguish between radiculopathies, plexopathies, and neuropathies, and clinch whether a neuropathy involves one or several nerves. However, a specific diagnosis cannot be made by this means.

To summarize, EMG examination may provide a guide to the time of onset of the lesion and to its chronicity, indicate whether the weakness has a neurogenic basis or not, and help to grade the severity and provide clues about dealing with the recovery (**Tables 2 and 3**).

INTRAOPERATIVE NERVE MONITORING

Recently, intraoperative recordings from peripheral nerves by techniques similar to those used in NCSs have been shown to be useful for early recognition and management of nerve insults during surgery. The intraoperative recordings have helped to identify individual nerves and determine whether they are in continuity, and identify the localization of the lesion to a specific site.[5,6] Continuous intraoperative nerve monitoring has been used in spine surgery to help predict and prevent neurologic complications.[7–10] Axillary nerve monitoring has been used during thermal capsulorrhaphy to prevent nerve injury.[11] Continuous nerve monitoring during shoulder anthroplasty has also been performed by Nagda and colleagues.[12] Monitoring was performed with the help of both transcranial electrical motor-evoked potentials (MEPs) and spontaneous EMG activity. No patient received regional anesthesia. A significant nerve event was defined by sustained neurotonic EMG activity or greater

Table 1
Peripheral nerve injury: ENMG recordings

| | Electromyography | | | | Response to Nerve Stimulation | |
| | | | Motor Unit Potentials | | | |
	Insertion Activity	Abnormal Spontaneous Activity	Number	Configuration	Proximal Stimulation	Distal Stimulation
Conduction Block						
Before recovery	Unchanged	None	Reduced	Normal	Reduced	Normal
<7 d	—	—	—	—	Reduced	—
>7 d	—	—	—	—	Reduced	—
During recovery	Unchanged	None	Increases to normal	Normal	Increases to normal	Normal
Axonal Degeneration						
Before recovery	—	—	Reduced	Normal	—	—
<7 d	Increased	None	—	—	Reduced	Normal
>7 d	Increased	Present	—	—	Reduced	Reduced
During recovery	Normalizes	Lessens	Increases to normal	Abnormal	Increases to normal	Increases to normal

Table 2
Time course of neurophysiologic recordings after nerve damage associated with regional anesthesia

Early <1 Week	Late >1 Week
Motor Nerve Fibers	
• MEP (latency and amplitudes) are altered	• MEP remain altered
• mNCS (amplitudes) remains unchanged	• mNCS (amplitudes) deteriorate within 7–10 d
• F-waves are altered	• F-waves remain altered
• EMG reveals reduced activation	• EMG reveals increasing signs of denervation and reduced activation
Sensory Nerve Fibers	
• SSEP (latency and amplitudes) are altered after regional anesthesia is vanished	• SSEP remain altered
• sNCS remain unchanged	• sNCS amplitude becomes altered
Sudomotor Fibers	
• SSR are altered after regional anesthesia vanishes	• SSR remain altered

Abbreviations: EMG, electromyography; MEP, motor-evoked potential; sNCS, sensory nerve conduction study; SSEP, somatosensory-evoked potential; SSR, sudomotor skin response.

than 50% amplitude reduction in the transcranial electrical MEPs from 1 or more muscles (or both). Of 30 patients, 17 (57%) had nerve alerts during the course of surgery. A total of 30 nerve alerts were recorded in the 30 patients. In 47% there were combined alerts with multiple nerves involved that pointed to dysfunction at the level of the trunk (or cord). Five events were related to impending injury of the musculocutaneous nerve, 3 with the ulnar nerve and 2 limited to the ulnar nerve. Nerve dysfunction occurred at any time during surgery from exposure until closure. Removal of the retractors without repositioning the arm did not result in a return to the baseline nerve signal in any case. When this was associated with repositioning of the operated arm to the neutral position, return of the nerve signal occurred in 77% of the events. Of the patients who did not have a complete return of function, 3 had evidence of an axillary nerve injury and 1 had a plexopathy involving the lower trunk. However, in all cases complete recovery was observed by 6 months postoperatively. This well-conducted and documented investigation emphasizes the crucial role of positioning and stretching of the nerves, conditions necessary for the performance of surgery, to explain the

Table 3
Pathophysiology of nerve damage

Pathophysiology	Key Neurophysiologic Finding
Neuropraxia (conduction block)	MEP/SSEP become altered, but NCS and EMG remain normal over time
Axonotmesis (axonal degeneration)	MEP/SSEP are altered whereas s/mNCS and EMG show signs of partial damage
Neurotmesis (nerve degeneration)	All neurophysiologic recordings become completely abolished

Abbreviations: EMG, electromyography; MEP, motor-evoked potential; NCS, nerve conduction study; SSEP, somatosensory-evoked potential; s/mNCS, sensory/motor nerve conduction study.

development of postoperative nerve damage. The importance of these factors in this setting has also been clearly demonstrated by Kwaan and Rappaport.[13]

Continuous perioperative nerve monitoring is not a common practice in surgery, except for major spine surgery. One may wonder whether, for example, patients at risk of nerve damage (previous shoulder surgery and limited preoperative external rotation)[12] undergoing shoulder arthroplasty would not benefit from this monitoring. Further studies are needed to clarify this issue. It is reasonable to believe that continuous nerve monitoring, especially transcranial electrical MEPs may help to better define the mechanism of perioperative nerve injury and thereby lead to improve surgical technique.[14]

HOW TO PROCEED

Both NCSs and EMG provide useful information for anesthesiologists in cases of new motor or sensory deficit after surgery. The examinations help to determine the basis of any deficit, to localize the responsible lesion, and to define its severity and prognosis. However, they do not help to define the direct cause of the damage, although the location and age of the injury in addition to the underlying pathologic process (demyelination changes or axon loss) may help to distinguish between different causes. The timing and the order of examinations to be performed is summarized in **Fig. 1**. MRI or ultrasonography of the puncture area should be performed to exclude a compression such as a hematoma. If this investigation is negative, one should not forget to investigate the surgical site for the same reason. If the sudomotor test is available, it should be performed to exclude an early CRPS type I or II. This syndrome has been shown to occur in some cases very early after surgery.[2] Conduction studies and EMG should be performed within the first days after the damage has been assessed to exclude a previous unknown subclinical polyneuropathy. In this case, ENMG of the contralateral side is indicated. Somatosensory and MEPs should also be performed early after the injury. These are particularly indicated if proximal damage (close to the spine) is suspected.

TREATMENT

To date, there is unfortunately no proven pharmacologic treatment to increase or effectively stimulate peripheral nerve regeneration. Regeneration is a long process occurring at a rate of 1 mm per day. Adjusted physiotherapy to prevent muscle atrophy and preserve range of motion of paralyzed joints as well as the treatment of neuropathic pain still remain the cornerstones of medical treatment. Recent understandings have demonstrated that peripheral nerve repair is not easily achieved to a high functional level although there is a much higher extent of neuron survival, neuritis outgrowth, and increased remyelination in the peripheral nervous system than in the central nervous system. Regenerating motor nerve fibers have the potential to arborize and travel across nerve stumps as induced by lesions but they need to be directed to avoid misconnections. In this context, functional electric stimulation (FES) has been shown in experimental studies to have positive effects on motor nerve fibers and alpha motorneurones.[15–17] This technique may be considered a potential means to improve peripheral nerve repair and functional restoration. To date, there is evidence that well-controlled FES is effective to build muscle volume and prevent extensive muscle atrophy. However, the impact on neural repair that can be immediately translated into functional improvement remains speculative. As an integral part of the treatment, the anesthesiologist should be in close contact with the patient during this long recovery process.

SUMMARY

The incidence of neurologic damage after regional anesthesia is rare. However, this complication may have dramatic consequences for the patient because its recovery may take several months. As nerve conduction studies and electromyography are the cornerstones of investigations in cases of postblock deficit, it is mandatory for the anesthesiologist performing regional anesthesia to have a basic understanding of these tests to discuss the cause with the surgeon and inform the patient about the prognosis.

REFERENCES

1. Capdevila X, Pirat P, Bringuier S, et al. Continuous peripheral nerve blocks in hospital wards after orthopedic surgery: a multicenter prospective analysis of the quality of postoperative analgesia and complications in 1,416 patients. Anesthesiology 2005;103:1035–45.
2. Borgeat A, Ekatodramis G, Kalberer F, et al. Acute and nonacute complications associated with interscalene block and shoulder surgery: a prospective study. Anesthesiology 2001;95:875–80.
3. Chaudhry V, Cornblath DR. Wallerian degeneration in human nerves: serial electrophysiological studies. Muscle Nerve 1992;15:687–93.
4. Blumenthal S, Borgeat A, Maurer K, et al. Preexisting subclinical neuropathy as a risk factor for nerve injury after continuous ropivacaine administration through a femoral nerve catheter. Anesthesiology 2006;105:1053–6.
5. Brown WF, Veitch J. AAEM minimonograph #42: intraoperative monitoring of peripheral and cranial nerves. Muscle Nerve 1994;17:371–7.
6. Daube JR, Harper CM. Monitoring peripheral nerves during surgery, Neuromuscular function and disease: basic, clinical, and electrodiagnostic aspects, vol. 2. Philadelphia: Saunders; 2002. p. 1857–65.
7. Fan D, Schwartz DM, Vaccaro AR, et al. Intraoperative neurophysiologic detection of iatrogenic C5 nerve root injury during laminectomy for cervical compression myelopathy. Spine (Phila Pa 1976) 2002;27:2499–502.
8. Hilibrand AS, Schwartz DM, Sethuraman V, et al. Comparison of transcranial electric motor and somatosensory evoked potential monitoring during cervical spine surgery. J Bone Joint Surg Am 2004;86:1248–53.
9. Nuwer MR, Dawson EG, Carlson LG, et al. Somatosensory evoked potential spinal cord monitoring reduces neurologic deficits after scoliosis surgery: results of a large multicenter survey. Electroencephalogr Clin Neurophysiol 1995;96: 6–11.
10. Schwartz DM, Wierzbowski LR, Fan D, et al. Surgical neurophysiologic monitoring. In: Vaccaro AR, Betz RR, Zeidman SM, editors. Principles and practice of spine surgery. Philadelphia: Mosby; 2003. p. 115–26.
11. Esmail AN, Getz CL, Schwartz DM, et al. Axillary nerve monitoring during arthroscopic shoulder stabilization. Arthroscopy 2005;21:665–71.
12. Nagda SH, Rogers KJ, Sestokas AK, et al. Peripheral nerve function during shoulder arthroplasty using intraoperative nerve monitoring. J Shoulder Elbow Surg 2007;16:S2–8.
13. Kwaan JH, Rappaport I. Postoperative brachial plexus palsy. A study on the mechanism. Arch Surg 1970;101:612–5.

14. Jellish WS, Blakeman B, Warf P, et al. Somatosensory evoked potential monitoring used to compare the effect of three asymmetric sternal retractors on brachial plexus function. Anesth Analg 1999;88:292–7.
15. Udina E, Furey M, Busch S, et al. Electrical stimulation of intact peripheral sensory axons in rats promotes outgrowth of their central projections. Exp Neurol 2008;210:238–47.
16. Lu MC, Tsai CC, Chen SC, et al. Use of electrical stimulation at different current levels to promote recovery after peripheral nerve injury in rats. J Trauma 2009;67: 1066–72.
17. Gordon T, Amirjani N, Edwards DC, et al. Brief post-surgical electrical stimulation accelerates axon regeneration and muscle reinnervation without affecting the functional measures in carpal tunnel syndrome patients. Exp Neurol 2009;219: 258–65.

Complications of Regional Anesthesia and Acute Pain Management

Terese T. Horlocker, MD

KEYWORDS

- Perioperative nerve injuries • Regional anesthesia
- Neurologic deficits • Surgical complications

Perioperative nerve injuries have long been recognized as a complication of regional anesthesia. Fortunately, severe or disabling neurologic complications rarely occur. Risk factors contributing to neurologic deficit after regional anesthesia include neural ischemia (hypothetically be related to the use of vasoconstrictors or prolonged hypotension), traumatic injury to the nerves during needle or catheter placement, infection, and choice of local anesthetic solution.[1-4] In addition, postoperative neurologic injury due to pressure from improper patient positioning or from tightly applied casts or surgical dressings, as well as surgical trauma, are often attributed to the regional anesthetic.[5] Lynch and colleagues[6] reported a 4.3% incidence of neurologic complications following total shoulder arthroplasty. The neurologic deficit localized to the brachial plexus in 75% of affected patients. Importantly, the level of injury occurred most commonly at the upper and middle nerve trunks—the level at which an interscalene block is performed, making it impossible to determine the cause of the nerve injury (surgical vs anesthetic). Patient factors such as body habitus or a preexisting neurologic condition may also contribute.[7-9] For example, the incidence of peroneal nerve palsy following total knee replacement is increased in patients with significant valgus or a preoperative neuropathy and the severity is increased in patients receiving epidural analgesia (**Table 1**).[10,11] The safe conduct of neuraxial anesthesia involves knowledge of the large patient surveys as well as individual case reports of neurologic deficits following neural blockade. Prevention of complications, along with early diagnosis and treatment are important factors in management of regional anesthetic risks.

INCIDENCE OF NEUROLOGIC COMPLICATIONS

Although severe or disabling neurologic complications are rare, recent epidemiologic series suggest the frequency of some serious complications is increasing. A

Department of Anesthesiology, Mayo Clinic, 200 First Street SW, Rochester, MN, 55905, USA
E-mail address: horlocker.terese@mayo.edu

Anesthesiology Clin 29 (2011) 257–278
doi:10.1016/j.anclin.2011.04.006
1932-2275/11/$ – see front matter © 2011 Published by Elsevier Inc.

anesthesiology.theclinics.com

Table 1
Risk profile for peroneal nerve palsy after total knee arthroplasty

Risk Factor	Peroneal Palsy (n = 8)	No Peroneal Nerve Palsy (n = 353)
Age (y)	64 ± 10	69 ± 10
Valgus (degrees)	13 ± 5[a]	9 ± 7
Tourniquet time (min)	141 ± 52[a]	103 ± 28
Neurologic condition	4[a]	30
Anesthetic technique		
General	3	112
Spinal	1	67
Epidural	4	174
Epidural analgesia	4[b]	104
Postoperative bleeding	3[a]	4

[a] P<0.05.
[b] Although postoperative epidural analgesia was not a risk factor for peroneal nerve palsy, all cases of peroneal nerve palsy with motor deficits occurred in patients with postoperative epidural analgesia.
Adapted from Horlocker TT, Cabanela ME, Wedel DJ. Does postoperative epidural analgesia increase the risk of peroneal nerve palsy after total knee arthroplasty? Anesth Analg 1994;79: 495–500; with permission.

prospective survey in France recently evaluated the incidence and characteristics of serious complications related to regional anesthesia.[2] Participating anesthesiologists kept a log of all cases and detailed information of serious complications occurring during or after regional anesthetics. All patients with a neurologic deficit lasting more than 2 days were examined by a neurologist; patients with cauda equina syndrome were evaluated with a CT scan to rule out compressive causes. A total of 103,730 regional anesthetics, were performed over 5 months. The incidence of cardiac arrest and neurologic complications was significantly higher after spinal anesthesia than other types of regional procedures (**Table 2**). Neurologic recovery was complete within 3 months in 29 of 34 patients with deficits. In 12 of 19 cases of radiculopathy after spinal anesthesia, and in all cases of radiculopathy after epidural or peripheral block, needle placement was associated with either paresthesia during needle insertion, or pain with injection. In all cases, the radiculopathy had the same topography as the associated paresthesia. The investigators concluded that needle

Table 2
Complications related to regional anesthesia

Technique	Cardiac Arrest	Death	Seizure	Neurologic Injury
Spinal (N = 40,640)	26 (3.9–8.9)	6 (0.3–2.7)	0 (0–0.9)	24 (3.5–8.3)
Epidural (N = 30,413)	3[a] (0.2–2.9)	0 (0–1.2)	4 (0.4–3.4)	6[a] (0.4–3.6)
Peripheral Blocks (N = 21,278)	3[b] (0.3–4.1)	1 (0–2.6)	16[c] (3.9–11.2)	4[c] (0.5–4.8)
IV Regional (N = 11,229)	0 (0–3.3)	0 (0–3.3)	3 (0.5–7.8)	0 (0–3.3)

Data presented are number and (95% confidence interval).
[a] Epidural versus spinal (P<.05).
[b] Peripheral nerve blocks versus spinal (P<.05).
[c] Peripheral nerve blocks versus epidural (P<.05).
Data from Auroy Y, Narchi P, Messiah A, et al. Serious complications related to regional anesthesia: results of a prospective survey in France. Anesthesiology 1997;7:479–86.

trauma and local anesthetic neurotoxicity were the causes of most neurologic complications. In a follow-up investigation performed with similar methodology 5 years later, the investigators reported a slight decrease of neurologic complications related to regional anesthetic technique.[12]

An epidemiologic study evaluating severe neurologic complications after neuraxial block conducted in Sweden between 1990 and 1999 reported some disturbing trends.[13] During the 10 year study period, approximately 1,260,000 spinal and 450,000 epidural (including 200,000 epidural blocks for labor analgesia) were performed. A total of 127 serious complications were noted, including spinal hematoma (33), cauda equina (32), meningitis (29), and epidural abscess (13). The nerve damage was permanent in 85 patients. Complications occurred more often after epidural than spinal blockade, and were different in character; cauda equina syndrome, spinal hematoma, and epidural abscess were more likely to occur after epidural block, whereas meningitis was more often associated with a spinal technique. Undiagnosed spinal stenosis (detected during evaluation of the new neurologic deficits) was a risk factor for cauda equina syndrome and paraparesis with both techniques. In the 18 cases of cauda equina syndrome following spinal anesthesia, 5% hyperbaric lidocaine was administered in eight cases, while bupivacaine (hyperbaric or isobaric) was the local anesthetic in 11 cases. This large series suggests that the incidence of severe anesthesia-related complications is not as low as previously reported. Moreover, since serious complications were noted to occur even in the presence of experienced anesthesiologists, continued vigilance in patients undergoing neuraxial anesthesia is warranted.

For example, Cheney and colleagues[14] examined the American Society of Anesthesiologists (ASA) Closed Claims database to determine the role of nerve damage following regional-pain block or general anesthesia in malpractice claims filed against anesthesia care providers. Of the 4,183 claims reviewed, 670 (16%) were for anesthesia-related nerve injury, including 189 claims involving the lumbosacral roots (105 claims) or spinal cord (84 claims); spinal cord injuries were the leading cause of claims for nerve injury that occurred in the 1990s, whereas injuries to the ulnar nerve or brachial plexus were more common previously. In addition, lumbosacral nerve root injuries having identifiable causes were associated predominantly with a regional (compared with general) anesthetic technique (92%), and were related to paresthesias during needle or catheter placement or pain during injection of local anesthetic. Major factors associated with spinal cord injury were blocks for chronic pain management and systemic anticoagulation in the presence of neuraxial block. A more recent ASA Closed Claims analysis of the 1005 cases of regional anesthesia claims from 1980 to 1999, reported that the majority of neuraxial complications associated with regional anesthesia claims resulted in permanent neurologic deficits.[15] Hematoma was the most common cause of neuraxial injuries and the majority of these cases were associated with either an intrinsic or an iatrogenic coagulopathy; 89% of patients had a permanent deficit. Conversely, complications caused by meningitis or abscess were more likely to be temporary. In a subset comparison of obstetric versus nonobstetric neuraxial anesthesia claims, obstetrics had a higher proportion of claims with low-severity and temporary injuries.

SPINAL CORD AND ROOT INJURY FROM NEURAXIAL NEEDLE AND CATHETER PLACEMENT

Direct needle or catheter-induced trauma rarely results in permanent or severe neurologic injury. A retrospective study of 4,767 spinal anesthetics noted the presence of a paresthesia during needle placement in 298 (6.3%) of patients. Importantly, four of the six patients with a persistent paresthesia postoperatively complained of a paresthesia during needle placement, identifying elicitation of a paresthesia as a risk factor for a persistent paresthesia.[16] As previously noted, in the series by Auroy and colleagues,[2] two-thirds of the patients with neurologic complications experienced pain during needle placement or injection of local anesthetic. In all cases, the neurologic deficit had the same distribution as the elicited paresthesia. It is unknown whether clinicians should abandon the procedure if a paresthesia is elicited (rather than repositioning the needle), in an effort to decrease the risk of nerve injury. This decision is complicated by the series of conus medullaris injuries following spinal (three cases) or combined spinal-epidural (four cases) anesthesia with a pencil point needle reported by Reynolds.[1] All seven patients complained of pain on needle insertion (only one noted pain on injection) and suffered damage to more than a single nerve root. In all patients, the anesthesiologist believed needle placement to have occurred at or below L2-3. A syrinx was noted on MRI in six cases suggesting intracord injection was the cause of the deficits. Cases of cord damage from needle insertion were also reported in the series by Auroy and colleagues[12] and Moen and colleagues.[13] Importantly, in all cases, the proceduralist had presumed the level of insertion to be below L1. These cases support the recommendation to insert needles below L3 to reduce the risk of direct needle trauma.[1,17]

The passage and presence of an indwelling catheter into the subarachnoid or epidural space presents an additional source of direct trauma. However, there is a lower frequency of persistent paresthesia or radiculopathy following epidural techniques, which are typically associated with (epidural) catheter placement, compared with single injection spinal anesthesia.[2,12,13] Although the incidence of neurologic complications associated with thoracic epidural techniques has historically been judged to be higher than that of lumbar placement, Giebler and colleagues[18] noted only a 0.2% incidence of postoperative radicular pain in 4185 patients undergoing thoracic epidural catheterization; all cases were responsive to catheter removal.

NERVE INJURY FROM PLEXUS-PERIPHERAL NEEDLE AND CATHETER PLACEMENT

Many anesthesiologists intentionally elicit a paresthesia during the performance of peripheral regional techniques. Although the elicitation of a paresthesia may represent direct needle trauma and increase the risk of persistent paresthesia associated with regional anesthesia, there are no clinical studies that definitively prove or refute the theory.[19–23] Selander and colleagues[21] reported a "higher" incidence of postoperative nerve injury in patients where a paresthesia was sought during axillary block (2.8%) compared with those undergoing a perivascular technique (0.8%). However, the difference was not statistically significant. Importantly, 40% of patients in the perivascular group reported unintentional paresthesias during the procedure, demonstrating the difficulty with standardization of technique and analysis of neural injury. Postoperative neurologic deficits ranged from slight hypersensitivity to severe paresis, and persisted from 2 weeks to greater than 1 year. In a prospective study using a variety of regional anesthetic approaches including paresthesia, transarterial, and nerve stimulator techniques, Urban and Urquhart[23] noted that mild paresthesias were common the day after surgery, occurring after 9% of interscalene blocks and after 19% of axillary blocks. At 2 weeks the incidence had decreased significantly, with near complete resolution noted at 4 weeks. Stan and colleagues[22] reported a 0.2% incidence of neurologic complications after axillary blocks performed with the transarterial approach. However, vascular complications such as transient arterial spasm, unintentional vascular injection, and hematoma formation occurred in 1.4% of patients.

Theoretically, localization of neural structures with a nerve stimulator would allow a high success rate without increasing the risk of neurologic complications, but this has not been formally evaluated. Fanelli and colleagues[19] prospectively evaluated 3996 patients undergoing sciatic-femoral, axillary, and interscalene blocks using a multiple injection, nerve stimulator technique. During the first month after surgery, 69 patients (1.7%) developed neurologic dysfunction; recovery was complete in all but one in 4 to 12 weeks. (This frequency is similar to that reported using a paresthesia technique). The only variable associated with neurologic injury was tourniquet inflation pressure greater than 400 mm Hg. Use of a nerve stimulator does not prevent intraneural injection. Indeed, serious neurologic injury has been reported following uneventful brachial plexus block using a nerve stimulator technique.[24,25] Equally interesting are the cases in which apparent intraneural injection did not result in neurologic injury.[26,27]

The use of ultrasound as a technique for neural localization continues to gain popularity and application. However, a superior efficacy and safety compared with other techniques has not been consistently demonstrated. For example, a recent systematic review (including both randomized control trials and case series) reported that use of ultrasound does not consistently improve the success of regional anesthesia versus most other techniques. However, ultrasound was not inferior for efficacy, did not increase risk, and offers other potential patient-oriented benefits.[20,28]

Currently, no compelling evidence exists to endorse a single technique as superior with respect to success rate or incidence of complications.[20] Needle gauge, type (short vs long bevel), and bevel configuration may also influence the degree of nerve injury, although the findings are conflicting and there are no confirmatory human studies (**Box 1**).[20,29,30]

Box 1
Recommendations for limiting peripheral nerve injury

- There are no animal or human data to support the superiority of one nerve localization technique—paresthesia, nerve stimulation, ultrasound—over another with regards to reducing the likelihood of nerve injury.

- Animal data have linked high injection pressures to subsequent fascicular injury, but there are no human data that confirm or refute the effectiveness of injection pressure monitoring for limiting nerve injury.

- There are no human data to support the superiority of one local anesthetic or additive over another with regard to reducing the likelihood of neurotoxicity.

- Patients with diseased or previously injured nerves (eg, diabetes mellitus, severe peripheral vascular disease, or chemotherapy) may theoretically be at increased risk for block-related nerve injury. Although isolated case reports have described new or progressive neurologic deficits after regional anesthetic techniques in patients with multiple sclerosis or previous exposure to chemotherapy, clinical experience can neither refute nor confirm these concerns. Based on limited animal data, consideration may be given to avoiding local anesthetics that are more potent, reducing local anesthetic doses and/or concentration, and avoiding or limiting vasoconstrictive additives in these patients.

- If damage to protective tissue barriers such as the perineurium is suspected from an abnormally painful paresthesia or pain on injection of local anesthetic, further injection should be halted immediately, and the needle repositioned. Consideration may be given to aborting the block procedure to avoid further deposition of local anesthetic and additive.

From Neal JM, Bernards CM, Hadzic A, et al. ASRA practice advisory on neurologic complications in regional anesthesia and pain medicine. Reg Anesth Pain Med 2008;33:404–15; with permission.

The potential added risk of neurologic complications resulting from placement of a plexus or peripheral nerve catheter remains undefined.[31] Although difficulty during catheter insertion may lead to vessel puncture, tissue trauma and bleeding, significant complications are uncommon and permanent sequelae are rare. In a recent prospective study involving 1,416 patients with continuous catheters, there were 12 patients (0.84%) experiencing serious adverse events and 3 (0.21%) patients had neurologic lesions attributed to the continuous peripheral nerve catheter.[32]

LOCAL ANESTHETIC TOXICITY

Neurologic complications after neuraxial anesthesia may be a direct result of local anesthetic toxicity. There is both laboratory and clinical evidence that local anesthetic solutions are potentially neurotoxic and that the neurotoxicity varies among local anesthetic solutions.[4,33–35] Neurotoxicity is dependent on Pka, lipid solubility, protein binding and potency. In histopathologic, electrophysiologic, and neuronal cell models, lidocaine and tetracaine appear to have a greater potential for neurotoxicity than bupivacaine at clinically relevant concentrations.[36] Additives such as epinephrine and bicarbonate may also affect neurotoxicity. The presence of a preexisting neurologic condition may predispose the nerve to the neurotoxic effects of local anesthetics.[9,33]

Although most local anesthetics administered in clinical concentrations and doses do not cause nerve damage, prolonged exposure, high dose, and/or high concentrations of local anesthetic solutions at the spinal roots may result in permanent neurologic deficits.[37] For example, cauda equina syndrome has been reported after single dose and continuous spinal anesthesia, intrathecal injection during intended epidural anesthesia, and repeated intrathecal injection after failed spinal block with lidocaine.[2,4,38] Presumably, injection (and/or reinjection) results in high concentrations of local anesthetic within a restricted area of the intrathecal space and causes neurotoxic injury. In the study by Auroy and colleagues,[2] 75% of the neurologic complications after uneventful (atraumatic) spinal anesthesia occurred in patients who received hyperbaric lidocaine, including one patient who received 350 mg over 5 hours with a 5% lidocaine infusion. Drasner[39] has recommended a maximum dose of 60 mg of lidocaine and the avoidance of epinephrine to prolong lidocaine spinal anesthesia. In addition, many clinicians recommend the use of isobaric solutions during continuous spinal techniques to reduce the risk of nonuniform distribution within the intrathecal space. Attention to patient positioning, total local anesthetic dose, and careful neurologic examination (evaluating for preferential sacral block) will assist in the decision to inject additional local anesthetic in the face of a patchy or failed block (**Box 2**).[40]

2-Chloroprocaine was introduced nearly 50 years ago as a local anesthetic for epidural administration. However, concern for neurotoxicity emerged 2 decades ago with a series of eight cases of neurologic injury associated with the use of Nesacaine-CE, a chloroprocaine solution containing the antioxidant sodium bisulfite. In all cases, the injury occurred after a large volume of anesthetic solution intended for the epidural space was accidentally administered intrathecally. Subsequent laboratory investigations evaluating the toxic contributions of 2-chloroprocaine, bisulfite, epinephrine, and pH reported that the commercial solution of 3% chloroprocaine (containing 0.2% sodium bisulfite, pH 3) produced irreversible block, but exposure to the same solution buffered to pH 7.3 resulted in complete recovery.[41] It was assumed that bisulfite was the source of neurotoxicity and that solutions that were bisulfite-free were safe for intrathecal use. More recently, these experiments were repeated with a more appropriate animal model and yielded different results: nerve

---

Box 2
Recommendations for anesthetic administration after a "failed spinal"

- Aspiration of cerebrospinal fluid (CSF) should be attempted before and after injection of anesthetic.

- Sacral dermatomes should always be included in an evaluation of the presence of a spinal block.

- If CSF is aspirated after anesthetic injection, it should be assumed that the local anesthetic has been delivered into the subarachnoid space; total anesthetic dosage should be limited to the maximum dose a clinician would consider reasonable to administer in a single injection.

- If an injection is repeated, the technique should be modified to avoid reinforcing the same restricted distribution (eg, alter patient position or switch to a local anesthetic of different baricity).

- If CSF cannot be aspirated after injection, repeat injection of a full dose of local anesthetic should not be considered unless careful sensory examination (conducted after sufficient time for development of sensory anesthesia) reveals no evidence of block.

From Drasner K. Local anesthetic neurotoxicity: clinical injury and strategies that may minimize risk. Reg Anesth Pain Med 2002;27:576–80; with permission.

---

injury scores were greater after administration of plain chloroprocaine compared with those of chloroprocaine containing bisulfite. These findings suggest clinical deficits associated with unintentional intrathecal injection of chloroprocaine likely resulted from a direct effect of the anesthetic, not the preservative. In addition, the data suggest that bisulfite can actually reduce neurotoxic damage induced by intrathecal local anesthetic.[42] Although recent clinical and volunteer studies[43] have not reported neurologic symptoms following spinal anesthesia with low-dose 2-chloroprocaine (30–40 mg), the laboratory evidence for toxicity warrants a cautious approach until additional toxicity data are available.

Transient Neurologic Symptoms

Transient neurologic symptoms (TNS) were first formally described in 1993. Schneider and colleagues[44] reported four cases of severe radicular back pain occurring after resolution of hyperbaric lidocaine spinal anesthesia. All four patients had undergone surgery in the lithotomy position. No sensory or motor deficits were detected on examination, and the symptoms resolved spontaneously within several days. Multiple laboratory and clinical studies have been performed in an attempt to define the causes, clinical significance, and risk factors associated with TNS. However, our understanding remains incomplete.

The incidence of TNS has ranged between 0% and 37%,[45–47] and is dependent on anesthetic, surgical, and probably undefined patient factors. A large, multicenter, epidemiologic study involving 1863 patients was recently performed to identify potential risk factors for TNS.[48] The incidence of TNS with lidocaine (11.9%) was significantly higher than that with tetracaine (1.6%) or bupivacaine (1.3%). The pain was described as severe in 30% of patients and resolved within a week in over 90% of cases. Outpatient status, obesity, and lithotomy position also increase the risk of TNS for patients who receive lidocaine. This suggests that the risk of TNS is high among outpatients in the lithotomy position (24.3%) and low for inpatients having surgery in positions other than lithotomy (3.1%). However, these variables were not risk factors with tetracaine or bupivacaine. The investigators also reported that neither gender, age, history of back pain or neurologic disorder, lidocaine dose or concentration, spinal needle or size, aperture direction, nor addition of epinephrine increased the risk of TNS (**Box 3**). These findings were confirmed in a systematic review of TNS.[49]

The high frequency of TNS with lidocaine spinal anesthesia has resulted in a search for a safe and effective alternative. The intrathecal administration of 2-chloroprocaine is under reconsideration due to the concern regarding toxicity, as previously mentioned. Mepivacaine may be a suitable substitute. In a series of 1273 patients undergoing spinal or combined spinal-epidural anesthesia, TNS occurred in only 78 (6.4%; 95% CI 5.1%–8%).[50]

The causes and clinical significance of TNS are unknown. Recent studies suggest local anesthetic toxicity, although the mechanism may not be identical to that of cauda equina syndrome.[51] Although many anesthesiologists believe that the reversible radicular pain is on one side of a continuum leading to irreversible cauda equina syndrome, there are no data to support this concept. It is important to distinguish between factors associated with serious neurologic complications, such as cauda equina syndrome, and transient symptoms when making recommendations for the clinical management of patients. For example, increasing the concentration or dose of lidocaine and adding epinephrine increases the risk of irreversible neurotoxicity, but has little effect on the risk of TNS. Therefore, the clinician must determine the appropriate intrathecal solution, including adjuvants, given the surgical duration and intraoperative position for each individual patient.

NEURAL ISCHEMIA

Local anesthetic solutions have varied effects on spinal cord blood flow. For example, lidocaine and tetracaine either maintain or increase blood flow, whereas bupivacaine and levobupivacaine result in a decrease.[52–55] The addition of epinephrine or phenylephrine results in a further decrease. However, in laboratory investigations, the alterations in blood flow are not accompanied by changes in histology or behavior.

Box 3
Factors that did not increase the risk of developing TNS after lidocaine spinal anesthesia

- Gender
- Age (<60 yr vs 60+ yr)
- Preexisting neurologic disorder or back pain
- Needle type (Quincke vs pencil point)
- Needle size (22 gauge vs 24–25 gauge vs 26–27 gauge)
- Bevel direction during injection (caudad vs cephalad vs LATERAL)
- Lidocaine dose (<50 mg vs 51–74 mg vs >75 mg)
- Intrathecal epinephrine
- Intrathecal opioid
- Intrathecal dextrose
- Paresthesia during needle placement

Data from Freedman JM, Li DK, Drasner K, et al. Transient neurologic symptoms after spinal anesthesia: an epidemiologic study of 1,863 patients. Anesthesiology 1998;89:633–41.

Likewise, large clinical studies have failed to identify the use of vasoconstrictors as a risk factor for temporary or permanent deficits. Most presumed cases of vasoconstrictor-induced neurologic deficits have been reported as single case reports, often with several other risk factors present.[2,56]

Peripheral nerves have a dual blood supply consisting of intrinsic endoneural vessels and extrinsic epineural vessels. A reduction or disruption of peripheral nerve blood flow may result in neural ischemia. Intraneural injection of volumes as small as 50 to 100 μL may generate intraneural pressures that exceed capillary perfusion pressure for as long as 10 minutes and thus cause neural ischemia.[57] Endoneural hematomas have also been reported after intraneural injection.[30] Epineural blood flow is also responsive to adrenergic stimuli.[58,59] The use of local anesthetic solutions containing epinephrine theoretically may produce peripheral nerve ischemia, especially in patients with microvascular disease.[3,33]

Finally, the addition of vasoconstrictors may potentiate the neurotoxic effects of local anesthetics. In a laboratory model, it was determined that the neurotoxicity of intrathecally administered lidocaine was increased by the addition of epinephrine.[60] A recent investigation by Sakura and colleagues[61] noted the addition of phenylephrine increased the risk of TNS in patients undergoing tetracaine spinal anesthesia (although no patient had sensory or motor deficits). However, the actual risk of significant neurologic ischemia causing neurologic compromise in patients administered local anesthetic solutions containing vasoconstrictors appears to be very low.

HEMORRHAGIC COMPLICATIONS

The actual incidence of neurologic dysfunction resulting from hemorrhagic complications associated with neuraxial blockade is unknown; however, recent epidemiologic studies suggest the incidence is increasing. In a review of the literature between 1906 and 1994, Vandermeulen and colleagues[62] reported 61 cases of spinal hematoma associated with epidural or spinal anesthesia. In 87% of patients, a hemostatic abnormality or traumatic or difficult needle placement was present. More than one risk factor was present in 20 of 61 cases. Importantly, although only 38% of patients had partial or good neurologic recovery, spinal cord ischemia tended to be reversible in patients who underwent laminectomy within 8 hours of onset of neurologic dysfunction.

The need for prompt diagnosis and intervention in the event of a spinal hematoma was also demonstrated in two reviews of the ASA Closed Claims database involving claims related to nerve injury.[14,15] Cheney and colleagues[14] examined the claims of nerve injury associated with general or regional block between 1990 and 1999 and noted that spinal cord injuries were the leading cause of claims in the 1990s. Furthermore, spinal hematomas accounted for nearly half of the spinal cord injuries. Patient care was rarely judged to have met standards due to delay in the diagnosis, and resultant poor outcome. Consequently, the median payment was very high. A more recent in-depth analysis of the claims related to nerve injury following regional anesthesia between 1980 and 1999 reported 36 spinal hematomas, associated mainly with vascular or orthopedic surgical procedures. Three-fourths of patients had evidence of a preexisting or iatrogenic coagulation abnormality.[15] Over half the patients received intravenous heparin during a vascular surgical or diagnostic procedure, often in combination with other medications that impair coagulation. Consistent with Vandermeulen and colleagues,[62] the presenting symptom was increased motor block (83% of cases), rather than back pain (25% of cases). Importantly, the presence of postoperative numbness or weakness was typically attributed to local anesthetic effect rather than spinal cord ischemia, which delayed the diagnosis. Although the symptoms were noted typically on the first postoperative day, often 24 hours or more elapsed before diagnosis. There were permanent deficits in 90% of patients.

It is impossible to conclusively determine risk factors for the development of spinal hematoma in patients undergoing neuraxial blockade solely through review of the case series, which represent only patients with the complication and do not define those who underwent uneventful neuraxial analgesia. However, large inclusive surveys that evaluate the frequencies of complications (including spinal hematoma), as well as identify subgroups of patients with higher or lower risk, enhance risk stratification. Moen and colleagues[13] investigated serious neurologic complications among 1,260,000 spinal and 450,000 epidural blocks performed in Sweden over 10 years. Twenty-four of the 33 spinal hematomas occurred in the last 5 years of the decade surveyed. Of the 33 spinal hematomas, 24 occurred in females and 25 were associated with an epidural technique. A coagulopathy (existing or acquired) was present in 11 patients; two of these patients were parturients with hemolysis, elevated liver enzymes, and low platelets (HELLP) syndrome. Pathology of the spine was present in six patients. The presenting complaint was typically lower extremity weakness. Only 5 of 33 patients recovered neurologically (due to delay in the diagnosis or intervention). These demographics, risk factors, and outcomes confirm those of previous series. However, the methodology allowed for calculation of frequency of spinal hematoma among patient populations. For example, the risk associated with epidural analgesia in women undergoing childbirth was significantly less (1 in 200,000) than that in elderly women undergoing knee arthroplasty (1 in 3600, $P<.0001$). Likewise, women undergoing hip fracture surgery under spinal anesthesia had an increased risk of spinal hematoma (1 in 22,000) compared with all patients undergoing spinal anesthesia (1 in 480,000).

Overall, these series suggest that the risk of clinically significant bleeding varies with age (and associated abnormalities of the spinal cord or vertebral column), the presence of an underlying coagulopathy, difficulty during needle placement, and an indwelling neuraxial catheter during sustained anticoagulation (particularly with unfractionated, standard, or low-molecular- weight heparin [LMWH]); perhaps in a multifactorial manner. They also consistently demonstrate the need for prompt diagnosis and intervention.

Plexus and Peripheral Blockade in the Anticoagulated Patient

Although spinal hematoma is the most significant hemorrhagic complication of regional anesthesia due to the catastrophic nature of bleeding into a fixed and noncompressible space, the associated risk following plexus and peripheral techniques remains undefined. The most significant study involving the risk of hemorrhagic complications associated with peripheral blocks included 670 patients undergoing continuous lumbar plexus blocks who were anticoagulated with warfarin.[63] Nearly all catheters were removed on the second postoperative day. At the time of catheter removal, 36% of patients had an international normalized ratio (INR) greater than 1.4. One case of local bleeding was noted in a patient with a corresponding INR of 3.0, which was treated with local pressure.

The Third American Society of Regional Anesthesia and Pain Medicine Practice Advisory on Regional Anesthesia and Antithrombotic Therapy reviewed all published cases of clinically significant bleeding or bruising after plexus or peripheral techniques.[64] In all patients with neurodeficits, neurologic recovery was complete within 6 to 12 months. Thus, although bleeding into a neurovascular sheath may result in significant decreases in hematocrit, the expandable nature of peripheral site may decrease the chance of irreversible neural ischemia. Of the 13 patients with bleeding complications following peripheral or plexus block in patients without anticoagulation, 5 were serious and required hospitalization, transfusion and/or surgical intervention (including one emergency tracheostomy after traumatic stellate block). Two of the 13 complications occurred after lumbar sympathetic or paravertebral techniques. There were also 13 cases of hemorrhagic complications associated with peripheral or plexus block in patients receiving antithrombotic therapy preblock and/or post-block. Twelve of these complications were serious, including one death due to massive hemorrhage following lumbar sympathetic block in a patient receiving clopi-dogrel. In all but one patient, hospitalization was complicated and prolonged. Nearly half of the patients received enoxaparin within 24 hours of the technique. Although this may implicate LWMH, it is also representative of the orthopedic patients who undergo lower extremity block and subsequently undergo thromboprophylaxis. Three of the patients were receiving nonsteroidal antiinflammatory drugs only.

This series of 26 patients is insufficient to make definitive recommendations. However, trends are evolving which may assist with patient management. For example, these cases suggest that significant blood loss, rather than neural deficits may be the most serious complication of non-neuraxial regional techniques in the anticoagulated patient. In addition, hemorrhagic complications following the deep plexus or peripheral techniques (eg, lumbar sympathetic, lumbar plexus, and paravertebral), particularly in the presence of antithrombotic therapy, are often serious and a source of major patient morbidity. Consequently, for patients undergoing deep plexus or peripheral block, it is recommended that guidelines regarding neuraxial techniques be similarly applied.

The decision to perform spinal or epidural anesthesia or analgesia and the timing of catheter removal in a patient receiving thromboprophylaxis should be made on an individual basis—weighing the small, though definite, risk of spinal hematoma with the benefits of regional anesthesia for a specific patient. Alternative anesthetic and analgesic techniques exist for patients considered to be at an unacceptable risk. The patient's coagulation status should be optimized at the time of spinal or epidural needle or catheter placement, and the level of anticoagulation must be carefully moni-tored during the period of epidural catheterization (**Table 3**). It is important to note that patients respond with variable sensitivities to anticoagulant medications. Indwelling catheters should not be removed in the presence of a significant coagulopathy, as this appears to significantly increase the risk of spinal hematoma.[13,62,65] In addition, communication between clinicians involved in the perioperative management of patients receiving anticoagulants for thromboprophylaxis is essential to decrease the risk of serious hemorrhagic complications. The patient should be closely moni-tored in the perioperative period for signs of cord ischemia. If spinal hematoma is sus-pected, the treatment of choice is immediate decompressive laminectomy.

INFECTIOUS COMPLICATIONS

Bacterial infection of the central neuraxis may present as meningitis or cord compres-sion secondary to abscess formation. Possible risk factors include underlying sepsis, diabetes, depressed immune status, steroid therapy, localized bacterial colonization or infection, and chronic catheter maintenance. The infectious source for meningitis and epidural abscess may result from distant colonization or localized infection with subsequent hematogenous spread and CNS invasion. The anesthetist may also trans-mit microorganisms directly into the CNS by needle or catheter contamination through a break in aseptic technique or passage through a contiguous infection. An indwelling neuraxial catheter, though aseptically sited, may be colonized with skin flora and conse-quently serve as a source for ascending infection to the epidural or intrathecal space.

Table 3 Neuraxial anesthesia and anticoagulation	
Warfarin	Discontinue chronic warfarin therapy 4–5 days before spinal procedure and evaluate INR. INR should be within the normal range at time of procedure to ensure adequate levels of all vitamin K-dependent factors. Postoperatively, daily INR assessment with catheter removal occurring with INR <1.5
Antiplatelet medications	No contraindications with aspirin or other NSAIDs. Thienopyridine derivatives (clopidogrel and ticlopidine) should be discontinued 7 d and 14 d, respectively, before procedure. GP IIb/IIIa inhibitors should be discontinued to allow recovery of platelet function before procedure (8 h for tirofiban and eptifibatide, 24–48 h for abciximab).
Thrombolytics/fibrinolytics	There are no available data to suggest a safe interval between procedure and initiation or discontinuation of these medications. Follow fibrinogen level and observe for signs of neural compression.
LMWH	Delay procedure at least 12 h from the last dose of thromboprophylaxis LMWH dose. For "treatment" dosing of LMWH, at least 24 h should elapse before procedure. LMWH should not be administered within 24 h after the procedure. Indwelling epidural catheters should be maintained with caution and only with once daily dosing of LMWH and strict avoidance of additional hemostasis altering medications, including ketorolac.
Unfractionated SQ heparin	There are no contraindications to neuraxial procedure if total daily dose is less than 10,000 units. For higher dosing regimens, manage according to intravenous heparin guidelines.
Unfractionated IV heparin	Delay needle/catheter placement 2–4 hours after last dose, document normal aPTT. Heparin may be restarted 1 h following procedure. Sustained heparinization with an indwelling neuraxial catheter associated with increased risk; monitor neurologic status aggressively.

Abbreviations: aPTT, activated partial thromboplastin time; GP IIb/IIIa, platelet glycoprotein receptor IIb/IIIa inhibitors; INR, international normalized ratio; LMWH, low-molecular-weight heparin; NSAIDs, nonsteroidal antiinflammatory drugs.

Data from Horlocker TT, Wedel DJ, Benzon H, et al. Regional anesthesia in the anticoagulated patient: defining the risks (the second ASRA Consensus Conference on Neuraxial Anesthesia and Anticoagulation). Reg Anesth Pain Med 2003;28:172–97; and Horlocker TT, Wedel DJ. Anticoagulation and neuraxial blockade: historical perspective, anesthetic implications, and risk management. Reg Anesth Pain Med 1998;23:129–34.

Historically, the frequency of serious CNS infections such as arachnoiditis, meningitis, and abscess following spinal or epidural anesthesia was considered to be extremely low—cases were reported as individual cases or small series.[66,67] However, recent epidemiologic series from Europe suggest that the frequency of infectious complications associated with neuraxial techniques is increasing.[13,68,69] In a national study conducted from 1997 to 1998 in Denmark, Wang and colleagues[69] reported the incidence of epidural abscess after epidural analgesia was 1 in 1930 catheters. Patients with epidural abscess had an extended duration of epidural catheterization (median 6 days, range 3–31 days). In addition, the majority of the patients with epidural abscess were immunocompromised. Often the diagnosis was delayed; the time to first symptom to confirmation of the diagnosis was a median of 5 days. *Staphylococcus aureus* was isolated in 67% of patients. Patients without neurologic deficits were successfully treated with antibiotics, while those with deficits underwent surgical decompression, typically with only moderate neurologic recovery.

In the series by Moen and colleagues[13] there were 42 serious infectious complications. Epidural abscess occurred in 13 patients; 9 (70%) were considered immunocompromised as a result of diabetes, steroid therapy, cancer, or alcoholism. Six patients underwent epidural block for analgesia following trauma. The time from placement of the epidural catheter to first symptoms ranged from 2 days to 5 weeks (median 5 days). Although prevailing symptoms were fever and sever backache, 5 developed neurologic deficits. All seven positive cultures isolated *S aureus*. Overall neurologic recovery was complete in 7 of 12 patients. However, 4 of the 5 patients with neurologic symptoms did not recover. Meningitis was reported in 29 patients for an overall incidence of 1:53,000. A documented perforation of the dura (intentional or accidental) occurred in 25 of 29 cases. In the 12 patients in whom positive cultures were obtained, alpha-hemolytic streptococci (pathogens common to the oropharynx) were isolated in 11 patients and *S aureus* in 1.

These large epidemiologic studies represent new and unexpected findings regarding the demographics, frequency, causes, and prognosis of infectious complications following neuraxial anesthesia. Epidural abscess is most likely to occur in immunocompromised patients with prolonged durations of epidural catheterization. The most common causative organism is *S aureus*, which suggests the colonization and subsequent infection from normal skin flora as the pathogenesis. In addition, delays in diagnosis and treatment result in poor neurologic recovery, despite surgical decompression. Conversely, patients who develop meningitis following neuraxial blockade typically are healthy and have undergone uneventful spinal anesthesia. Furthermore, the series by Moen and colleagues[13] validates the findings of individual case reports of meningitis after spinal anesthesia—the source of the pathogen is mostly likely to be in the upper airway.[70]

Infectious complications may also occur after plexus and peripheral techniques. Indwelling catheters theoretically increase the risk of infectious complications. However, although colonization may occur, infection is rare.[32] Risk factors appear to be similar to those associated with neuraxial blockade and include duration of catheterization, compromised immune status, and absence of antibiotic prophylaxis.[32,71]

Aseptic Technique

Although previous publications have repeatedly recommended meticulous aseptic technique, only recently have standards for asepsis during the performance of regional anesthetic procedures been defined.[72,73] Hand washing remains the most crucial component of asepsis; gloves should be regarded as a supplement to—not a replacement of—hand washing.[74] The use of an antimicrobial soap reduces bacterial growth and reduces the risk of bacteria being released into the operative field should gloves become torn or punctured during the procedure. An alcohol-based antiseptic provides the maximum degree of antimicrobial activity and duration. Prior to washing, all jewelry (eg, rings, watches) should be removed; higher microbial counts have been noted in health care workers who do not routinely remove these items before hand washing. Sterile gloves protect not only patients from contamination, but also health care workers from blood-borne pathogens and are required by the Occupational Safety and Health Administration. Glove leaks are more likely to occur with vinyl compared with latex gloves (24% vs 2%), with contamination of the health care workers' hands noted following the leaks in 23% of cases.[75] Conversely, the use of gowns does not further reduce the likelihood of cross contamination in an intensive care unit setting compared with gloves alone. At this time, there are insufficient data to make recommendations regarding routine use for single injection or temporary neuraxial or peripheral catheter placement. However, placement of an indwelling permanent device, such as a spinal cord stimulator, warrants the same asepsis as a surgical procedure, including gowns, hats, and antibiotic pretreatment.[72,76] Surgical masks, initially considered a barrier to protect the proceduralist from patient secretions and blood, are now required by the Center for Disease Control[77] due to the increasing number of cases of post-spinal meningitis, many of which result from contamination of the epidural or intrathecal space with pathogens from the operator's buccal mucosa.[13,70,78]

Antiseptic solutions

Controversy still exists regarding the most appropriate and safe antiseptic solution for patients undergoing neuraxial and peripheral techniques. Povidone iodine and chlorhexidine gluconate (with or without the addition of isopropyl alcohol) have been most extensively studied.[79,80] In nearly all clinical investigations, the bactericidal effect of chlorhexidine was more rapid and more effective (extending its effect for hours following its application) than povidone iodine. The addition of isopropyl alcohol accelerates these effects. Chlorhexidine is effective against nearly all nosocomial yeasts and bacteria (gram-positive and gram-negative); resistance is extremely rare. It also remains effective in the presence of organic compounds, such as blood. It must be noted that chlorhexidine-alcohol labeling contains a warning against use as a skin preparation before lumbar puncture. The Food and Drug Administration has not formally approved chlorhexidine for skin preparation before lumbar puncture because of the lack of animal and clinical studies examining the neurotoxic potential of chlorhexidine—not because of the number of reported cases of nerve injury. Indeed, it is important to note that there are no cases of neurotoxicity with either chlorhexidine or alcohol.[72] Therefore, because of its superior effect, alcohol-based chlorhexidine solutions are considered the antiseptic of choice for skin preparation before any regional anesthetic procedure.[72,73]

REGIONAL BLOCK IN PATIENTS WITH PREEXISTING NEUROLOGIC DISORDERS

Patients with preexisting neurologic disease present a unique challenge to the anesthesiologist. The cause of postoperative deficits is difficult to evaluate, because neural injury may occur because of surgical trauma, tourniquet pressure, prolonged labor, improper patient positioning, or anesthetic technique. Progressive neurologic diseases such as multiple sclerosis may coincidentally worsen perioperatively, independent of the anesthetic method. The most conservative legal approach is to avoid regional anesthesia in these patients. However, high-risk patients, including those with significant cardiopulmonary disease, may benefit medically from regional anesthesia and analgesia. The decision to proceed with a regional anesthesia in these patients should be made on a case-by-case basis.

The presence of preexisting deficits, signifying chronic neural compromise, theoretically places these patients at increased risk for further neurologic injury. The presumed mechanism is a "double crush" of the nerve at two locations resulting in a nerve injury of clinical significance.[81] The double crush concept suggests that nerve damage caused by traumatic needle placement or local anesthetic toxicity during the performance of a regional anesthetic may worsen neurologic outcome in the presence of an additional patient factor or surgical injury.[8,9,11,82,83] Progressive neurologic diseases may also coincidentally worsen perioperatively, independent of the anesthetic method. If a regional anesthetic is indicated or requested, the patient's preoperative neurologic examination should be formally documented and the patient must be made aware of the possible progression of the underlying disease process (**Box 4**).[20]

Multiple Sclerosis

It is difficult to define the relative risk of neurologic complications in patients with pre-existing neurologic disorders who receive regional anesthesia; no controlled studies have been performed, and accounts of complications have appeared in the literature as individual case reports. Although laboratory studies have identified multiple risk

---

Box 4
Recommendations for performing regional anesthesia in patients with preexisting neurologic conditions

- Overall approach to patients with preexisting neurologic deficits
  - Patients with preexisting neurologic disease may be at increased risk of new or worsening injury regardless of anesthetic technique. When regional anesthesia is thought to be appropriate for these patients, modifying the anesthetic technique may minimize potential risk. Based on a moderate amount of animal data, such modifications may include using a less potent local anesthetic, minimizing local anesthetic dose, volume, and/or concentration, and avoiding or using a lower concentration of vasoconstrictive additives. Limited human data neither confirm nor refute these modifications.

- Preexisting peripheral neuropathy
  - Patients with chronic diabetes mellitus, severe peripheral vascular disease, multiple sclerosis, or previous exposure to chemotherapy (eg, cisplatin or vincristine) may have clinical or subclinical evidence of a preexisting peripheral neuropathy. Peripheral nerve block may theoretically increase the risk of new or progressive postoperative neurologic complications in these patients. However, existing data can neither confirm nor refute this theory in clinical practice. Under these clinical conditions, a careful risk-to-benefit assessment of regional anesthesia to alternative perioperative anesthesia and analgesia techniques should be considered.

- Preexisting CNS disorders
  - Definitive evidence indicating that neuraxial anesthesia or analgesia may increase the risk of new or progressive postoperative neurologic complications in patients with preexisting CNS disorders (eg, multiple sclerosis, postpolio syndrome) is lacking. However, under these clinical conditions, a careful risk-to-benefit assessment of regional anesthesia to alternative perioperative anesthesia and analgesia techniques should be considered.

- Spinal stenosis or mass lesions within the spinal canal
  - In patients with known severe spinal stenosis or mass lesions within the spinal canal, a careful risk-to-benefit assessment of regional anesthesia to alternative perioperative anesthesia and analgesia techniques should be considered. In these patients, high local anesthetic volume neuraxial techniques (eg, epidural anesthesia) may be associated with a higher risk of progressive mass effect when compared with low volume techniques (eg, spinal anesthesia).
  - For patients receiving neuraxial injection for treatment of pain (eg, cervical epidural injection of steroids via an interlaminar route), radiologic imaging studies such as computed tomography or magnetic resonance imaging should be used to assess the dimensions of the spinal canal, and this information should be considered in the overall risk-to-benefit analysis, as well as guiding the selection of the safest level for entry.

Adapted from Neal JM, Bernards CM, Hadzic A, et al. ASRA practice advisory on neurologic complications in regional anesthesia and pain medicine. Reg Anesth Pain Med 2008;3:404–15; with permission.

factors for the development of neurologic injury after regional anesthesia, clinical studies are lacking. Even less information is available for the variables affecting neurologic damage in patients with preexisting neurologic disease. The largest series of neuraxial anesthesia in the patient with a preexisting CNS condition involved 139 patients.[8] Postpolio syndrome and multiple sclerosis were the most common CNS disorders. The majority of patients had sensorimotor deficits at the time of block placement. There were no patients with new or worsening postoperative neurologic deficits when compared with preoperative findings (0.0%; 95% CI 0.0%–0.3%). The investigators concluded that the risks commonly associated with neuraxial block in patients with preexisting CNS disorders may not be as high as thought and that these conditions should not be an absolute contraindication to spinal or epidural techniques. Because multiple sclerosis is a disorder of the CNS, peripheral nerve blocks do not affect neurologic function and are considered appropriate anesthetic techniques. However, the clinician should be aware of the potential for the presence of an associated peripheral neuropathy (which exists in over 10% of patients).[84]

Diabetes Mellitus

A substantial proportion of diabetic patients report clinical symptoms of a neuropathy. However, a subclinical neuropathy may be present before the onset of pain, paresthesia, or sensory loss and may remain undetected without electrophysiologic testing showing typical slowing of nerve conduction velocity. The presence of underlying nerve dysfunction suggests that patients with diabetes may have a decreased requirement for local anesthetic. The diabetes-associated microangiopathy of nerve blood vessels decreases the rate of absorption, resulting in prolonged exposure to local anesthetic solutions. The combination of these two mechanisms may cause nerve injury with an otherwise safe dose of local anesthetic in diabetic patients. In a study examining the effect of local anesthetics on nerve conduction block and injury in diabetic rats, Kalichman and Calcutt[33] reported that the local anesthetic requirement is decreased and the risk of local anesthetic-induced nerve injury is increased in diabetes.

A recent retrospective review of 567 patients with a sensorimotor neuropathy or diabetic polyneuropathy who underwent neuraxial block evaluated the risk of neurologic complications. All patients had a single neurologic diagnosis; there were no coexisting spinal canal or CNS disorders.[9] The majority of patients had sensorimotor deficits at the time of surgery. Two (0.4%; 95% CI 0.1%–1.3%) patients experienced new or worsening postoperative neurologic deficits in the setting of uneventful neuraxial block and without surgical or positioning risk factors. In these patients, who had severe sensorimotor neuropathy preoperatively, it is likely the neuraxial technique contributed to the injury.

Spinal Stenosis and Lumbar Root Disease

Moen and colleagues[13] identified spinal stenosis as a risk factor for postoperative cauda equina syndrome and paraparesis. Importantly, deficits would often occur after uneventful neuraxial technique. These findings agree with those of a recent investigation that examined the overall success and neurologic complication rates among 937 patients with spinal stenosis or lumbar disc disease undergoing neuraxial block.[83] Two hundred seven patients had a history of prior spinal surgery before undergoing neuraxial block, although the majority were simple laminectomies or discectomies. Ten (1.1%; 95% CI 0.5%–2.0%) patients experienced new or progressive neurologic deficits when compared with preoperative findings. A surgical cause was presumed to be the primary cause in four of ten patients. The primary cause of the remaining six complications was judged nonsurgical (including anesthetic-related factors). The investigators concluded that patients with a history of preexisting spinal stenosis or lumbar radiculopathy are at increased risk of neurologic complications following neuraxial blockade. Because the cause of the complications is likely multifactorial, until the relative contribution of existing patient and potential surgical contributing factors is known, the decision to perform neuraxial blockade in these patients should be made cautiously.

In general, patients with preoperative neurologic deficits may undergo further nerve damage more readily from needle or catheter placement, local anesthetic systemic toxicity, and vasopressor-induced neural ischemia. Consequently, when feasible, dilute or less potent local anesthetic solutions should be used in order to decrease the risk of local anesthetic toxicity. Because epinephrine and phenylephrine also prolong the block and, therefore, neural exposure to local anesthetics, the appropriate concentration and dose of local anesthetic solutions must be thoughtfully considered.[20]

REGIONAL ANESTHESIA IN ANESTHETIZED ADULTS

The actual risk of neurologic complications in patients undergoing regional techniques while anesthetized or heavily sedated has not been formally evaluated. However, epidemiologic series report direct trauma and toxicity as the causes of most neurologic complications and have identified pain during needle placement or injection of local anesthetic as major risk factors.[2,12,14] Thus, performance of regional blocks while the patient is under general anesthesia theoretically increases the risk of perioperative neurologic complications, since these patients are unable to respond to the pain associated with needle- or catheter-induced paresthesias or intraneural injections. Despite these findings, there are few data to support these concerns. Cases are typically reported individually; no randomized study or large review has been performed to date.[24,25] Importantly, the apparent safety of performing regional techniques under general anesthesia that is demonstrated in the pediatric literature must be carefully interpreted. There are also medicolegal issues.

Peripheral and plexus blocks (compared with neuraxial techniques) may represent additional risk when performed on an anesthetized patient. The larger dose of local anesthetic given as a single bolus over a relatively short interval increases the risk of systemic toxicity, whereas heavy sedation or general anesthesia diminishes the patient's ability to report early signs of rising local anesthetic blood levels. In addition, although some peripheral techniques are performed as a field block, most require that the nerve or sheath be directly identified by eliciting a paresthesia or nerve stimulator response or by locating an adjacent vascular structure. However, the use of a nerve stimulator or ultrasound does not replace the patient's ability to respond to the pain of needle trauma or intraneural injection. Urmey and Stanton[85] performed interscalene blocks on patients who were not already medicated using paresthesia techniques with insulated (10 patients) and noninsulated (20 patients) needles. Paresthesias were elicited with the nerve stimulator power off. Upon elicitation of the paresthesia, the nerve stimulator was turned on and the amperage slowly increased to a maximum of 1.0 mA. Only 30% of patients exhibited any motor response. Benumof[24] reported four cases of permanent cervical spinal cord injury following interscalene block performed with the patient under general anesthesia or heavy sedation. In three cases, a nerve stimulator was used to localize the brachial plexus. These results suggest that since it is possible to have sensory nerve contact and not elicit a motor response, use of a nerve stimulator (and unpublished data associated with ultrasound guided blocks) does not protect the anesthetized patient from nerve injury.[20] Thus, the decision to perform a regional anesthetic on a heavily sedated or anesthetized patient should not be made indiscriminately.

SUMMARY

In conclusion, major complications after regional anesthetic techniques are rare, but can be devastating to the patient and the anesthesiologist. Prevention and management begin during the preoperative visit with a careful evaluation of the patient's medical history and appropriate preoperative discussion of the risks and benefits of the available anesthetic techniques. The decision to perform a regional anesthetic technique on an anesthetized patient must be made with care since these patients are unable to report pain on needle placement or injection of local anesthetic. Efforts should also be made to decrease neural injury in the operating room through careful patient positioning. Postoperatively, patients must be followed closely to detect potentially treatable sources of neurologic injury, including constrictive dressings, improperly applied casts, and increased pressure on neurologically vulnerable sites. New neurologic deficits should be evaluated promptly by a neurologist, or neurosurgeon, to formally document the patient's evolving neurologic status, arrange further testing or intervention, and provide long-term follow-up.[20]

REFERENCES

1. Reynolds F. Damage to the conus medullaris following spinal anaesthesia. Anaesthesia 2001;56:238–47.
2. Auroy Y, Narchi P, Messiah A, et al. Serious complications related to regional anesthesia: results of a prospective survey in France. Anesthesiology 1997;87:479–86.
3. Myers RR, Heckman HM. Effects of local anesthesia on nerve blood flow: studies using lidocaine with and without epinephrine. Anesthesiology 1989;71:757–62.
4. Rigler ML, Drasner K, Krejcie TC, et al. Cauda equina syndrome after continuous spinal anesthesia. Anesth Analg 1991;72:275–81.
5. Brull R, McCartney CJ, Chan VW, et al. Effect of transarterial axillary block versus general anesthesia on paresthesiae 1 year after hand surgery. Anesthesiology 2005;103:1104–5.
6. Lynch NM, Cofield RH, Silbert PL, et al. Neurologic complications after total shoulder arthroplasty. J Shoulder Elbow Surg 1996;5:53–61.
7. Warner MA, Warner DO, Harper CM, et al. Lower extremity neuropathies associated with lithotomy positions. Anesthesiology 2000;93:938–42.
8. Hebl JR, Horlocker TT, Schroeder DR. Neuraxial anesthesia and analgesia in patients with preexisting central nervous system disorders. Anesth Analg 2006;103:223–8.
9. Hebl JR, Kopp SL, Schroeder DR, et al. Neurologic complications after neuraxial anesthesia or analgesia in patients with preexisting peripheral sensorimotor neuropathy or diabetic polyneuropathy. Anesth Analg 2006;103:1294–9.
10. Horlocker TT, Cabanela ME, Wedel DJ. Does postoperative epidural analgesia increase the risk of peroneal nerve palsy after total knee arthroplasty? Anesth Analg 1994;79:495–500.
11. Horlocker TT, Hebl JR, Gali B, et al. Anesthetic, patient, and surgical risk factors for neurologic complications after prolonged total tourniquet time during total knee arthroplasty. Anesth Analg 2006;102:950–5.

12. Auroy Y, Benhamou D, Bargues L, et al. Major complications of regional anesthesia in France: the SOS Regional Anesthesia Hotline Service. Anesthesiology 2002;97:1274–80.
13. Moen V, Dahlgren N, Irestedt L. Severe neurological complications after central neuraxial blockades in Sweden 1990–1999. Anesthesiology 2004;101:950–9.
14. Cheney FW, Domino KB, Caplan RA, et al. Nerve injury associated with anesthesia: a closed claims analysis. Anesthesiology 1999;90:1062–9.
15. Lee LA, Posner KL, Domino KB, et al. Injuries associated with regional anesthesia in the 1980s and 1990s: a closed claims analysis. Anesthesiology 2004;101:143–52.
16. Horlocker TT, McGregor DG, Matsushige DK, et al. A retrospective review of 4767 consecutive spinal anesthetics: central nervous system complications. Anesth Analg 1997;84:578–84.
17. Reynolds F. Logic in the safe practice of spinal anaesthesia. Anaesthesia 2000;55:1045–6.
18. Giebler RM, Scherer RU, Peters J. Incidence of neurologic complications related to thoracic epidural catheterization. Anesthesiology 1997;86:55–63.
19. Fanelli G, Casati A, Garancini P, et al. Nerve stimulator and multiple injection technique for upper and lower limb blockade: failure rate, patient acceptance, and neurologic complications. Study Group on Regional Anesthesia. Anesth Analg 1999;88:847–52.
20. Neal JM, Bernards CM, Hadzic A, et al. ASRA practice advisory on neurologic complications in regional anesthesia and pain medicine. Reg Anesth Pain Med 2008;33:404–15.
21. Selander D, Edshage S, Wolff T. Paresthesiae or no paresthesiae? Nerve lesions after axillary blocks. Acta Anaesthesiol Scand 1979;23:27–33.
22. Stan TC, Krantz MA, Solomon DL, et al. The incidence of neurovascular complications following axillary brachial plexus block using a transarterial approach. A prospective study of 1,000 consecutive patients. Reg Anesth 1995;20:486–92.
23. Urban MK, Urquhart B. Evaluation of brachial plexus anesthesia for upper extremity surgery. Reg Anesth 1994;19:175–82.
24. Benumof JL. Permanent loss of cervical spinal cord function associated with interscalene block performed under general anesthesia. Anesthesiology 2000;93:1541–4.
25. Passannante AN. Spinal anesthesia and permanent neurologic deficit after interscalene block. Anesth Analg 1996;82:873–4.
26. Bigeleisen PE. Nerve puncture and apparent intraneural injection during ultrasound-guided axillary block does not invariably result in neurologic injury. Anesthesiology 2006;105:779–83.
27. Borgeat A. Regional anesthesia, intraneural injection, and nerve injury: beyond the epineurium. Anesthesiology 2006;105:647–8.
28. Liu SS, Ngeow JE, Yadeau JT. Ultrasound-guided regional anesthesia and analgesia: a qualitative systematic review. Reg Anesth Pain Med 2009;34:47–59.
29. Rice AS, McMahon SB. Peripheral nerve injury caused by injection needles used in regional anaesthesia: influence of bevel configuration, studied in a rat model. Br J Anaesth 1992;69:433–8.
30. Selander D, Dhuner KG, Lundborg G. Peripheral nerve injury due to injection needles used for regional anesthesia. An experimental study of the acute effects of needle point trauma. Acta Anaesthesiol Scand 1977;21:182–8.
31. Motamed C, Bouaziz H, Mercier FJ, et al. Knotting of a femoral catheter. Reg Anesth 1997;22:486–7.

32. Capdevila X, Pirat P, Bringuier S, et al. Continuous peripheral nerve blocks in hospital wards after orthopedic surgery: a multicenter prospective analysis of the quality of postoperative analgesia and complications in 1,416 patients. Anesthesiology 2005;103:1035–45.
33. Kalichman MW, Calcutt NA. Local anesthetic-induced conduction block and nerve fiber injury in streptozotocin-diabetic rats. Anesthesiology 1992;77:941–7.
34. Ready LB, Plumer MH, Haschke RH, et al. Neurotoxicity of intrathecal local anesthetics in rabbits. Anesthesiology 1985;63:364–70.
35. Myers RR, Sommer C. Methodology for spinal neurotoxicity studies. Reg Anesth 1993;18:439–47.
36. Hodgson PS, Neal JM, Pollock JE, et al. The neurotoxicity of drugs given intrathecally (spinal). Anesth Analg 1999;88:797–809.
37. Drasner K, Sakura S, Chan VW, et al. Persistent sacral sensory deficit induced by intrathecal local anesthetic infusion in the rat. Anesthesiology 1994;80:847–52.
38. Drasner K, Rigler ML, Sessler DI, et al. Cauda equina syndrome following intended epidural anesthesia. Anesthesiology 1992;77:582–5.
39. Drasner K. Lidocaine spinal anesthesia: a vanishing therapeutic index? Anesthesiology 1997;87:469–72.
40. Drasner K. Local anesthetic neurotoxicity: clinical injury and strategies that may minimize risk. Reg Anesth Pain Med 2002;27:576–80.
41. Gissen A, Datta S, Lambert D. The chloroprocaine controversy. II. Is chloroprocaine neurotoxic? Reg Anesth 1984;9:135–44.
42. Taniguchi M, Bollen AW, Drasner K. Sodium bisulfite: scapegoat for chloroprocaine neurotoxicity? Anesthesiology 2004;100:85–91.
43. Yoos JR, Kopacz DJ. Spinal 2-chloroprocaine for surgery: an initial 10-month experience. Anesth Analg 2005;100:553–8.
44. Schneider M, Ettlin T, Kaufmann M, et al. Transient neurologic toxicity after hyperbaric subarachnoid anesthesia with 5% lidocaine. Anesth Analg 1993;76:1154–7.
45. Pollock JE, Liu SS, Neal JM, et al. Dilution of spinal lidocaine does not alter the incidence of transient neurologic symptoms. Anesthesiology 1999;90:445–50.
46. Pollock JE, Neal JM, Stephenson CA, et al. Prospective study of the incidence of transient radicular irritation in patients undergoing spinal anesthesia. Anesthesiology 1996;84:1361–7.
47. Hampl KF, Schneider MC, Ummenhofer W, et al. Transient neurologic symptoms after spinal anesthesia. Anesth Analg 1995;81:1148–53.
48. Freedman JM, Li DK, Drasner K, et al. Transient neurologic symptoms after spinal anesthesia: an epidemiologic study of 1,863 patients. Anesthesiology 1998;89:633–41.
49. Zaric D, Christiansen C, Pace NL, et al. Transient neurologic symptoms after spinal anesthesia with lidocaine versus other local anesthetics: a systematic review of randomized, controlled trials. Anesth Analg 2005;100:1811–6.
50. YaDeau JT, Liguori GA, Zayas VM. The incidence of transient neurologic symptoms after spinal anesthesia with mepivacaine. Anesth Analg 2005;101:661–5, table of contents.
51. Johnson ME, Uhl CB, Spittler KH, et al. Mitochondrial injury and caspase activation by the local anesthetic lidocaine. Anesthesiology 2004;101:1184–94.
52. Kozody R, Ong B, Palahniuk RJ, et al. Subarachnoid bupivacaine decreases spinal cord blood flow in dogs. Can Anaesth Soc J 1985;32:216–22.
53. Kozody R, Palahniuk RJ, Cumming MO. Spinal cord blood flow following subarachnoid tetracaine. Can Anaesth Soc J 1985;32:23–9.

54. Kozody R, Swartz J, Palahniuk RJ, et al. Spinal cord blood flow following subarachnoid lidocaine. Can Anaesth Soc J 1985;32:472–8.
55. Kristensen JD, Karlsten R, Gordh T. Spinal cord blood flow after intrathecal injection of ropivacaine: a screening for neurotoxic effects. Anesth Analg 1996;82: 636–40.
56. Dahlgren N, Tornebrandt K. Neurological complications after anaesthesia. A follow-up of 18,000 spinal and epidural anaesthetics performed over three years. Acta Anaesthesiol Scand 1995;39:872–80.
57. Selander D, Sjostrand J. Longitudinal spread of intraneurally injected local anesthetics. An experimental study of the initial neural distribution following intraneural injections. Acta Anaesthesiol Scand 1978;22:622–34.
58. Bouaziz H, Iohom G, Estebe JP, et al. Effects of levobupivacaine and ropivacaine on rat sciatic nerve blood flow. Br J Anaesth 2005;95:696–700.
59. Neal JM. Effects of epinephrine in local anesthetics on the central and peripheral nervous systems: neurotoxicity and neural blood flow. Reg Anesth Pain Med 2003;28:124–34.
60. Hashimoto K, Hampl KF, Nakamura Y, et al. Epinephrine increases the neurotoxic potential of intrathecally administered lidocaine in the rat. Anesthesiology 2001; 94:876–81.
61. Sakura S, Sumi M, Sakaguchi Y, et al. The addition of phenylephrine contributes to the development of transient neurologic symptoms after spinal anesthesia with 0.5% tetracaine. Anesthesiology 1997;87:771–8.
62. Vandermeulen EP, Van Aken H, Vermylen J. Anticoagulants and spinal-epidural anesthesia. Anesth Analg 1994;79:1165–77.
63. Chelly JE, Szczodry DM, Neumann KJ. International normalized ratio and prothrombin time values before the removal of a lumbar plexus catheter in patients receiving warfarin after total hip replacement. Br J Anaesth 2008;101:250–4.
64. Horlocker TT, Wedel DJ, Rowlingson JC, et al. Regional anesthesia in the patient receiving antithrombotic or thrombolytic therapy: American Society of Regional Anesthesia and Pain Medicine Evidence-Based Guidelines (Third Edition). Reg Anesth Pain Med 2010;35:64–101.
65. Horlocker T, Wedel DJ. Neuraxial blockade and low molecular weight heparin: balancing perioperative analgesia and thromboprophylaxis. Reg Anesth Pain Med 1998;23:164–77.
66. Baker AS, Ojemann RG, Swartz MN, et al. Spinal epidural abscess. N Engl J Med 1975;293:463–8.
67. Ready LB, Helfer D. Bacterial meningitis in parturients after epidural anesthesia. Anesthesiology 1989;71:988–90.
68. Ericsson M, Algers G, Schliamser SE. Spinal epidural abscesses in adults: review and report of iatrogenic cases. Scand J Infect Dis 1990;22:249–57.
69. Wang LP, Hauerberg J, Schmidt JF. Incidence of spinal epidural abscess after epidural analgesia: a national 1-year survey. Anesthesiology 1999;91:1928–36.
70. Schneeberger PM, Janssen M, Voss A. Alpha-hemolytic streptococci: a major pathogen of iatrogenic meningitis following lumbar puncture. Case reports and a review of the literature. Infection 1996;24:29–33.
71. Bergman BD, Hebl JR, Kent J, et al. Neurologic complications of 405 consecutive continuous axillary catheters. Anesth Analg 2003;96:247–52.
72. Hebl JR. The importance and implications of aseptic techniques during regional anesthesia. Reg Anesth Pain Med 2006;31:311–23.
73. Horlocker TT, Birnbach DJ, Connis RT, et al. Practice advisory for the prevention, diagnosis, and management of infectious complications associated with neuraxial

techniques: a report by the American Society of Anesthesiologists Task Force on infectious complications associated with neuraxial techniques. Anesthesiology 2010;112:530–45.

74. Saloojee H, Steenhoff A. The health professional's role in preventing nosocomial infections. Postgrad Med J 2001;77:16–9.

75. Olsen RJ, Lynch P, Coyle MB, et al. Examination gloves as barriers to hand contamination in clinical practice. JAMA 1993;270:350–3.

76. Rathmell JP, Lake T, Ramundo MB. Infectious risks of chronic pain treatments: injection therapy, surgical implants, and intradiscal techniques. Reg Anesth Pain Med 2006;31:346–52.

77. Available at: http://www.cdc.gov/hicpac/pdf/isolation/Isolation2007.pdf. Accessed April 1, 2011.

78. Trautmann M, Lepper PM, Schmitz FJ. Three cases of bacterial meningitis after spinal and epidural anesthesia. Eur J Clin Microbiol Infect Dis 2002;21:43–5.

79. Birnbach DJ, Stein DJ, Murray O, et al. Povidone iodine and skin disinfection before initiation of epidural anesthesia. Anesthesiology 1998;88:668–72.

80. Kinirons B, Mimoz O, Lafendi L, et al. Chlorhexidine versus povidone iodine in preventing colonization of continuous epidural catheters in children: a randomized, controlled trial. Anesthesiology 2001;94:239–44.

81. Upton AR, McComas AJ. The double crush in nerve entrapment syndromes. Lancet 1973;2:359–62.

82. Hebl JR, Horlocker TT, Pritchard DJ. Diffuse brachial plexopathy after interscalene block in a patient receiving cisplatin chemotherapy: the pharmacologic double crush syndrome. Anesth Analg 2001;92:249–51.

83. Hebl JR, Horlocker TT, Kopp SL, et al. Neuraxial blockade in patients with preexisting spinal stenosis, lumbar disk disease, or prior spine surgery: efficacy and neurologic complications. Anesth Analg 2010;111:1511–9.

84. Koff MD, Cohen JA, McIntyre JJ, et al. Severe brachial plexopathy after an ultrasound-guided single-injection nerve block for total shoulder arthroplasty in a patient with multiple sclerosis. Anesthesiology 2008;108:325–8.

85. Urmey WF, Stanton J. Inability to consistently elicit a motor response following sensory paresthesia during interscalene block administration. Anesthesiology 2002;96:552–4.

Unintentional Subdural Injection: A Complication of Neuraxial Anesthesia/ Analgesia

Nir Hoftman, MD

KEYWORDS

- Neuraxial anesthesia • Neuraxial complications
- Subdural anesthesia • Subdural catheter

Unintentional subdural catheterization with subsequent local anesthetic injection continues to pose an often poorly recognized challenge to the anesthesiologist. The increasing popularity and availability of thoracic epidural analgesia for postsurgical patients necessitates prompt recognition of potential complications arising from mal-positioned catheters. Although subarachnoid and intravenous injections are usually easily recognized, the diagnosis of subdural injection is often made in retrospect, or not at all. Two factors make the clinical diagnosis of subdural injection difficult: (1) highly variable clinical presentation, and (2) little public awareness of the entity. Thus, the goal of this article is to discuss the clinical presentation, diagnosis, and management of subdural injection to increase public awareness of this unusual phenomenon.

The spinal subdural space has been defined clinically as a potential space with a small amount of serous fluid contained within.[1] This anatomic definition arose from experience with cadaveric and surgical dissection, at which time the dura and arachnoid membranes are easily separated from one another. It was thus assumed that subdural catheterizations occur when the epidural or spinal needle is inserted past the epidural space, pierces the dura mater, and enters the subdural potential space, which then expands with injection of fluid.[2] A more recent experiment per-formed on fresh cadavers using electron microscopy seems to suggest, however,

Funding was provided by the UCLA Anesthesiology Department Research Committee.
The author has nothing else to disclose.
Department of Anesthesiology, University of California Los Angeles, 757 Westwood Boulevard, Mail Code 740330, Los Angeles, CA 90095-7403, USA
E-mail address: nhoftman@mednet.ucla.edu

Anesthesiology Clin 29 (2011) 279–290
doi:10.1016/j.anclin.2011.04.002
1932-2275/11/$ – see front matter © 2011 Elsevier Inc. All rights reserved.
anesthesiology.theclinics.com

that rather than a potential space, the subdural space is an iatrogenic dissection of the thecal membranes.[3] In fact, there seems to be a natural cleavage plain that can occur between the dura mater and arachnoid membrane, as these 2 structures are normally approximated together with sparse cellular and noncellular connective tissue. Furthermore, other cleavage planes can also occur within the matrix of the dura mater fibers. Therefore, subdural injections likely represent a heterogeneous group of "intradural" injections that create a dissection within the membranes, either at the dura-arachnoid interface or through the matrix of the dura proper.

The incidence of unintentional subdural injection during epidural catheterization is widely quoted in textbooks to be 0.82%. This figure, however, originated from a retrospective study that defined the entity clinically and did not use radiographic imaging to confirm the diagnosis.[4] Other smaller prospective studies performed by radiologists and anesthesiologists that did confirm subdural injection radiographically reported incidence rates of 7% to 11%.[5–7] To determine the true incidence of unintentional subdural catheterization, a large, prospective trial of epidural anesthesia/analgesia with radiographic imaging of all catheters would need to be performed.

The vast majority of reported cases of unintentional subdural catheterization occur unexpectedly, without any prior warning that the epidural placement was faulty. However, there is some evidence that the following risk factors may increase the likelihood of subdural catheterization: (1) catheterization following lumbar puncture, (2) catheterization following previous subdural injection, (3) epidural needle rotation before catheter insertion, and (4) technically difficult block placement.[6–10] It is assumed that the common denominator among all 4 of these actions is physical damage to the dura that increases the likelihood of subdural catheter placement.

CLINICAL PRESENTATION

The "classic" subdural blockade described in the original case reports presented with several key features: (1) excessive sensory blockade, (2) sympatholysis out of proportion to local anesthetic dose, and (3) variable motor blockade.[11] As more case reports were published, different clinical patterns emerged. Cases of respiratory distress, unconsciousness, and even cardiac arrest were reported.[12–14] Equally worrisome were case reports of unrecognized subdural catheters that behaved initially like normal epidurals only to deteriorate upon further injection, often leading to life-threatening scenarios.[13,15] Such sensational reports left the practitioners expecting all subdural injections to be excessive and dramatic. However, over the past 2 decades, numerous case reports of "atypical" subdural blockades were published. Rather than presenting with excessive blockade, these cases presented with unilateral, restricted, and even failed blocks.[16,17] Perhaps the most bizarre subdural cases were catheters presumed to be subarachnoid owing to free-flowing cerebrospinal fluid (CSF) upon aspiration that failed to deliver appreciable spinal blockade upon local anesthetic injection.[18]

Given the heterogeneous presentation of subdural local anesthetic injection, this author recently reviewed 70 cases of radiographically confirmed thoracic and lumbar subdural catheters so as to more accurately describe their clinical presentation.[19] Not surprisingly, most cases described a slow onset and excessive sensory blockade. However, a significant minority of cases described restricted, unilateral distribution of sensory blockade. The incidence of each significant finding among the 70 cases is summarized graphically in **Fig. 1**. Of note, findings such as "motor-sparing blockade," cardiovascular depression, and respiratory distress, which were previously described as "defining characteristics," were seen in fewer than half of cases.

Furthermore, the volume of local anesthetic injected into the catheter seemed unrelated to the extent of sensory blockade and cardiovascular depression seen. Thus, it seems that the "classic presentation" of subdural injection represented just one facet of this entity's multifaceted clinical presentation. Why does subdural injection, unlike epidural or subarachnoid injection, present so heterogeneously and unpredictably? Is there an anatomic correlate to the clinical presentation? Do extensive blocks represent dissection through the "zipperlike" dura-arachnoid interface while restricted blocks represent "intradural" contained injections? Such recently proposed theories seem logical, and are awaiting the introduction of more sophisticated imaging modalities for the ultimate proof.

DIAGNOSIS AND TREATMENT

Correct diagnosis of unintentional subdural injection begins with a high index of suspicion. Although no one sign or symptom can guarantee the diagnosis, specific combinations of signs and symptoms can be highly suggestive. The key to making the diagnosis is to recognize unusual clusters of signs and symptoms. Such "unlikely pairings" of mutually antagonistic clinical findings suggest the diagnosis. For instance, an extensive sensory blockade after a small local anesthetic dose suggests subarachnoid block, but paired with other findings, such as negative aspiration test, slow onset, motor sparing, or lack of cardiovascular depression, make for a most unusual block. At the other end of the spectrum, a narrow, restricted block is not unusual in epidural anesthesia, but one coupled with life-threatening hypotension and a very delayed onset is unusual as well.

To better assist the clinician at making the clinical diagnosis of subdural injection, this author has created a clinical algorithm based on data from 70 confirmed subdural cases (**Fig. 2**). The algorithm, set up as a clinical road map, begins with the clinician presuming the suspicious neuraxial catheter to be either "epidural" or "subarachnoid" depending on the feel during placement and presence or absence of CSF aspiration. The second step is defining the sensory blockade as extensive, normal, or restricted. Finally, the presence of at least one of several minor criteria for that category increases the likelihood that the catheter is located in the subdural space.

Once the clinical suspicion for subdural catheterization begins to mount, the decision of how to proceed must be made. First and foremost is whether to discontinue catheter use; this decision is often more complex than it would initially seem. Patients with well-placed epidural catheters can present with significant hypotension, high blocks, respiratory insufficiency, and even patchy, unilateral blocks. Correct management of such epidural catheters can lead to a safe and effective anesthetic/analgesic. On the other hand, subdural catheters are unpredictable and can lead to life-threatening clinical deterioration, possibly many hours after seemingly normal function. The mechanism of such instability is likely multifactorial and may include subdural catheter migration, progressive meningeal dissection, and even arachnoid rupture with subsequent subarachnoid drug overdose.[20,21] Also, "intradural" injection may trap local anesthetic in the neuraxis, leading to a delayed effect from this medication depot. For this reason, subdural catheters should not be used in clinical practice, especially in environments that are not tightly supervised, such as patient hospital rooms, as would be the case with postoperative analgesia.

Therefore, if a subdural catheter is suspected, the catheter tip position should be confirmed radiographically or the neuraxial technique should be abandoned. Three main imaging options exist: (1) anteroposterior and lateral plain films, (2) live action fluoroscopy, and (3) computed tomography (CT) epidurography. In all 3 cases, 3 to

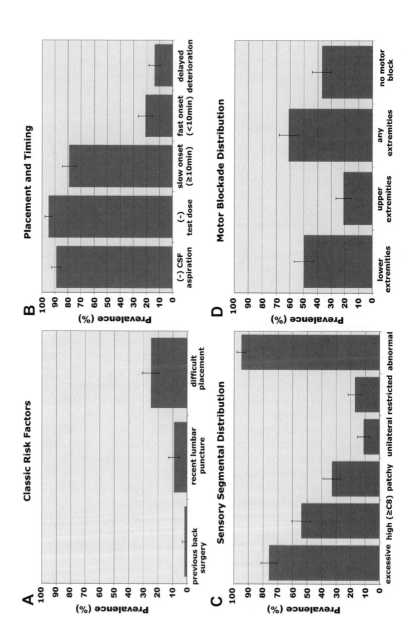

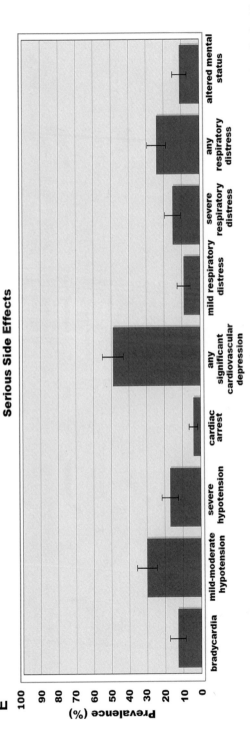

Fig. 1. Summary of the prevalence of numerous clinical characteristics of subdural injection. (A) highlights the prevalence of previously described "risk factors" for subdural cannulation. (B) describes characteristics of block placement and timing of clinical effect. (C) summarizes the sensory distribution of the segmental blockade. (D) illustrates the prevalence and distribution of motor blockade. (E) characterizes the prevalence of serious side effects reported as a result of unintentional subdural injection. (Reprinted from Hoffman N, Ferrante M. Diagnosis of unintentional subdural anesthesia/analgesia: analyzing radiographically proven cases to define the clinical entity and to develop a diagnostic algorithm. Reg Anesth Pain Med 2009;34(1):12–6; with permission.)

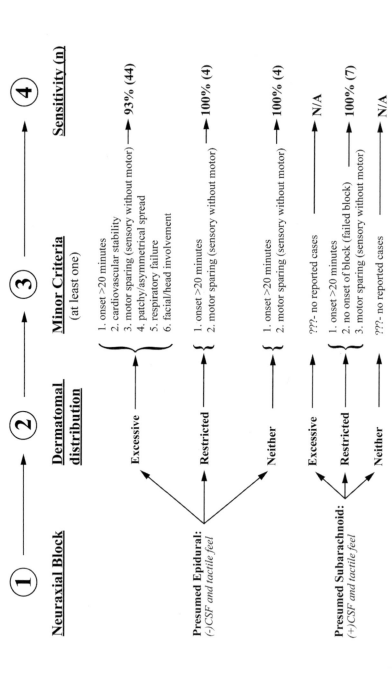

Fig. 2. A 4-step diagnostic algorithm designed to detect subdural injection. In the first step, the practitioner determines whether the neuraxial block in question is presumed to be epidural or subarachnoid based on the tactile feel at insertion and CSF absence or presence. The second step requires the provider to define the dermatomal spread as excessive, restricted, or neither. Minor criteria are then applied in step 3; at least one criterion is needed for the diagnosis to be made. The final step (4) displays the sensitivity of the test for diagnosing subdural injection in that subcategory and the number of cases from which it was derived. (*Reprinted from* Hoftman N, Ferrante M. Diagnosis of unintentional subdural anesthesia/analgesia: analyzing radiographically proven cases to define the clinical entity and to develop a diagnostic algorithm. Reg Anesth Pain Med 2009;34(1):12–6; with permission.)

6 mL of radiocontrast (such as Omnipaque 300, GE Healthcare, Princeton, NJ) should be injected just before the study. Plain films are the easiest and cheapest choice, but can be difficult to interpret, especially by non-neuroradiologists. Fluoroscopy gives the advantage of seeing the contrast flow into the space, which can be extremely useful in determining the catheter tip location in expert hands. Finally, CT epidurography is the costliest option, but allows for very high definition and tomographic axial cuts that delineate in great detail the contrast extension. Regardless of the option chosen, the importance of radiographic confirmation of catheter tip position before clinical use of an unusual neuraxial block cannot be overstated.

When faced with a clinically unstable patient with a suspected subdural injection, supportive care should be implemented immediately. Airway management and cardiovascular support are usually quickly effective, and even cases of intractable cardiovascular depression have been successfully managed with potent vasopressors and inotropes.[22,23] Of note, there are no cases of death from subdural injection reported in the literature, although many close calls have been described.

CASE-BASED LEARNING MODULES

Following are 3 actual case reports of patients who presented with unintentional subdural catheterization. These 3 cases vary widely and thus demonstrate the heterogeneity of the clinical presentation. All initially received thoracic epidural catheters before thoracic surgery that were to have been used for postoperative analgesia. Actual CT epidurograms are provided to illustrate the radiographic findings seen with subdural injection.

Case 1

A 70-year-old woman with a history of sarcoma was scheduled to undergo a video-assisted thoracoscopic surgery (VATS) resection of a solitary pulmonary nodule. Preoperatively, a thoracic epidural was easily and seemingly uneventfully placed at the T6-T7 interspace. Immediately upon the test dose injection (4 mL of 1.5% lidocaine with epinephrine), the patient complained of moderate to severe upper back and chest pain that waned and resolved within a few minutes. Fifteen minutes later the patient complained of numbness in her fingers. Neurological exam revealed dense bilateral T4-L2 sensory blockade, normal sensation between T1 and T4, and dense sensory loss in the C7-C8 dermatome (corresponding to the fourth and fifth fingers). Of note, despite this dense sensory blockade, there was no change in baseline motor strength, respiratory status, or blood pressure and heart rate.

Case discussion

Although pain or discomfort on epidural injection is occasionally seen, the combination of this unusual symptom and an excessive sensory block heightened suspicion for a subdural catheter. Looking at **Fig. 2**, this presentation fits into the following category: presumed epidural block with excessive sensory distribution. It also satisfies 3 minor criteria: (1) cardiovascular stability, (2) motor sparing, (3) patchy block. Although none of these criteria on their own would be diagnostic, this combination of "unlikely pairs" increases the suspicion that a subdural injection may have occurred. A high block with 1.5% lidocaine, were it to have been epidural or subarachnoid, should have demonstrated some cardiovascular depression and motor blockade. Furthermore, the patchy distribution that skipped dermatomes would be unusual for such blocks.

Given the clinical suspicion, the patient underwent CT epidurography using 6 mL of Omnipaque 180 radiocontrast. **Fig. 3** shows select cuts of this image that demonstrate contrast mostly in the subdural space with some extension into the epidural space as well.

Case 2

A 61-year-old woman who previously underwent orthotopic liver transplantation presented with idiopathic pulmonary fibrosis and was scheduled for a VATS lung biopsy. Following uneventful preoperative placement of a T6-T7 thoracic epidural, a 3-mL test dose (1.8% lidocaine with epinephrine and bicarbonate) was injected. Ten minutes after injection only a right-sided single dermatome (T7) of decreased sensation to cold stimulus was detected. A few minutes later the patient suddenly experienced a cardiovascular collapse and lost consciousness (blood pressure [BP] 50/30, heart rate [HR] 30). Following a very brief resuscitation with atropine 0.5 mg plus ephedrine 10 mg, the patient immediately regained consciousness as blood pressure and heart rate were restored. No change in the sensory exam was noted at that time. A full 40 minutes after the test dose, with the patient's hemodynamic status fully restored, a unilateral R-sided T6-T11 sensory block was noted.

Case discussion

Unilateral or restricted sensory blockade is not unusual during epidural anesthesia/ analgesia. However, life-threatening cardiovascular depression coupled with a nonexistent block is another example of "unlikely pairing" of signs and symptoms, and thus raises the possibility of a malpositioned catheter. Although subarachnoid injection should always be on the top of the differential in a patient who loses consciousness after epidural injection, the rapidity of the awakening after hemodynamic stabilization

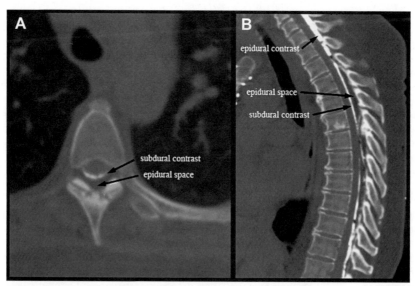

Fig. 3. CT epidurogram demonstrating radiocontrast mostly in the subdural compartment with some dye in the epidural space as well. (*A*) Axial CT cut at the midthoracic level demonstrating contrast (white rim posterior to the spinal cord) only in the subdural space. The epidural space (seen in black) is totally devoid of contrast. (*B*) Computer reconstructed lateral view demonstrating epidural contrast in the high thoracic spine and subdural contrast in the mid and lower thoracic spine.

and the complete absence of appreciable motor and sensory blockade raise the possibility of subdural injection. Plugging this case into the clinical roadmap places this patient in the presumed epidural category with restricted dermatomal distribution. The presence of one minor criterion (onset >20 minutes) further increases clinical suspicion that a subdural injection may have occurred.

Given this clinical suspicion, the patient underwent CT epidurography using 4 mL of Omnipaque 300 radiocontrast. **Fig. 4** shows select cuts of this image that demonstrate contrast mostly in the subdural space with some extension into the epidural space as well.

Case 3

A 60-year-old man with malignant mesothelioma underwent uneventful preoperative thoracic epidural placement (T7-T8) in anticipation of surgical tumor resection. A 3-mL 1.8% lidocaine with epinephrine and bicarbonate test dose was negative for intravenous and subarachnoid injection and failed to demonstrate any segmental sensory blockade after 15 minutes. A further 10 mL of the same solution was injected in divided doses. Fifteen minutes later (a full 30 minutes after the initial test dose), a bilateral T4-T10 dense sensory blockade to pin prick was noted. Blood pressure and heart rate were unchanged throughout this time (BP 150/80, HR 70).

General anesthesia was induced and the patient was positioned for thoracotomy. With commencement of the surgery (75 minutes after epidural injection), the patient became progressively hypotensive and bradycardic, with very poor responsiveness to vasopressors. Fluid resuscitation plus escalating doses of ephedrine,

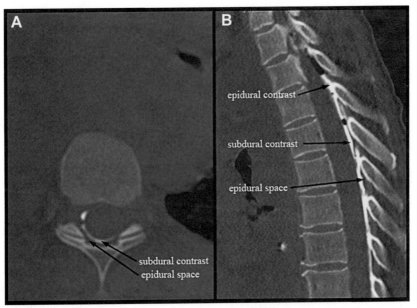

Fig. 4. CT epidurogram demonstrating radiocontrast mostly in the subdural compartment with some dye in the epidural space as well. (*A*) Axial CT cut at the low-thoracic level demonstrating contrast (white rim posterolateral to the spinal cord) confined to the subdural space. The epidural space (seen in black and very small in this patient) is totally devoid of contrast. (*B*) Computer-reconstructed lateral view demonstrating epidural contrast in the high thoracic spine and subdural contrast in the mid and lower thoracic spine.

phenylephrine, dopamine, epinephrine, and vasopressin were required to treat this intractable severe hypotension (BP 70/30). A pulmonary artery catheter was placed and a transesophageal echo exam was performed; both demonstrated a classic distributive shock picture composed of hyperdynamic circulation with low systemic vascular resistance. Anaphylaxis was presumed, given recent exposure to antibiotic, muscle relaxant, and latex gloves. Given the continuing cardiovascular instability, the operation was halted and a definitive diagnostic test was performed.

Case discussion

With the initial failure to elicit any sensory block after the test dose, this author suspected the catheter was malpositioned outside the neuraxis and thus a larger dose was administered to "prove the point." Surprisingly, a delayed onset block did emerge, the true extent of which will never be known, given that the patient underwent general anesthesia soon thereafter. Most baffling at the time was the lack of any change in heart rate and blood pressure. An hour later, when the patient was in profound distributive shock, it occurred to this author that a similar case report of subdural injection had been published. Although anaphylaxis still topped the differential, the combination of delayed onset, unusually stable blood pressure (initially), and later unusually unstable blood pressure led this author to temporarily halt the surgery and perform a CT epidurogram using 5 mL of Omnipaque 180. **Fig. 5** shows select cuts of this image that demonstrate contrast mostly in the subdural space with some extension into the epidural space as well.

Following CT epidurography, the patient returned to the operating room for completion of the operation, remaining hemodynamically stable for the remainder of the case.

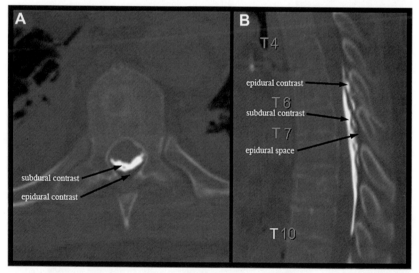

Fig. 5. CT epidurogram demonstrating radiocontrast mostly in the subdural compartment with some dye in the epidural space as well. (*A*) Axial CT cut at the midthoracic level demonstrating contrast (thick white collection posterior to the spinal cord) confined to the subdural space. The epidural space (seen in black) is totally devoid of contrast. (*B*) Computer-reconstructed lateral view demonstrating subdural contrast confined to the T6-T10 spinal levels. A small amount of epidural contrast is visible at T6-T7 near the entry point of the epidural catheter and likely represents efflux of dye from the subdural space into the epidural space.

The likelihood of both anaphylaxis and subdural injection seemed extremely unlikely and thus the distributive shock was ascribed solely to the subdural injection. Of note, the patient was rechallenged with multiple drugs and no further episodes of hypotension were noted. A normal serum tryptase level (which was available for examination 1 week later) ruled out anaphylaxis as a possible cause of the hypotension.

SUMMARY

Unintentional subdural injection during anesthesia/analgesia is presumed to be a rare event, although without large prospective trials, the true incidence will remain unknown. It is important to identify such cases, however, as failure to do so could lead to untoward complications and possible patient harm. The absolute anatomic mechanism that would explain the heterogeneous signs and symptoms of this entity has yet to be fully elucidated, although several researchers are working on better defining the anatomy and mechanism of subdural catheterization. For now, given the lack of a definitive set of diagnostic criteria, this author would recommend careful clinical observation coupled with use of the included clinical algorithm (see **Fig. 2**). Suspicious catheters should be discontinued or radiographic imaging should be performed to rule out subdural catheterization before continued clinical use of the neuraxial catheter.

REFERENCES

1. Brown DL. Spinal, epidural, and caudal anesthesia. In: Miller RD, editor. Anesthesia. 5th edition. Philadelphia: Churchill Livingstone; 2000. p. 1492–3.
2. Blobmerg RG. The lumbar subdural extraarachnoid space of humans: an anatomical study using spinaloscopy in autopsy cases. Anesth Analg 1987;66: 177–80.
3. Reina MA, De Leon Casasola O, Lopez A, et al. The origin of the spinal subdural space: ultrastructure findings. Anesth Analg 2002;94:991–5.
4. Lubenow T, Keh-Wong E, Kristof K, et al. Inadvertent subdural injection: a complication of an epidural block. Anesth Analg 1988;67:175–9.
5. Mehta M, Salmon N. Extradural block. Confirmation of the injection site by X-ray monitoring. Anaesthesia 1985;40:1009–12.
6. Collier CB. Accidental subdural injection during attempted lumbar epidural block may present as a failed or inadequate block: radiographic evidence. Reg Anesth Pain Med 2004;29:45–51.
7. Jones MD, Newton TH. Inadvertent extra-arachnoid injections in myelography. Radiology 1963;80:818–22.
8. Dominguez E, Latif O, Rozen D, et al. Subdural blood patch for the treatment of persistent leak after permanent intrathecal catheter implantation: a report of two cases. Pain Pract 2001;1:344–53.
9. Ischia S, Maffezzoli GF, Luzanni A, et al. Subdural extra-arachnoid neurolytic block in cervical pain. Pain 1982;14:347–54.
10. Duffy BL. Don't turn the needle! Anaesth Intensive Care 1993;21:328–30.
11. Collier C. Total spinal or massive subdural block? Anaesth Intensive Care 1982; 10:92–3.
12. Silva Costa-Gomes T, Montes A, Sanchez JC, et al. Cardiorespiratory arrest: a rare complication of subdural block. Rev Esp Anestesiol Reanim 2002;49: 108–11.

13. Forrester DJ, Mukherji SK, Mayer DC, et al. Dilute infusion for labor, obscure subdural catheter, and life-threatening block at cesarean delivery. Anesth Analg 1999;89:1267–8.
14. Rowbottom SJ, Kong AS, Chan M, et al. Subdural block. Anaesth Intensive Care 1993;21:132–3.
15. Haughton AJ, Chalkiadis GA. Unintentional paediatric subdural catheter with oculomotor and abducens nerve palsies. Paediatr Anaesth 1999;9:543–8.
16. Paech MJ. A most unusual subdural block. Anaesth Intensive Care 1988;16:488–90.
17. Mocan M, Gamulin Z, Klopfenstein CE, et al. Accidental catheterization of the subdural space: a complication of continuous spinal anesthesia and continuous peridural anesthesia. Can J Anaesth 1989;36:708–12.
18. Cohen CA, Kallos T. Failure of spinal anesthesia due to subdural catheter placement. Anesthesiology 1972;37:352–3.
19. Hoftman NH, Ferrante FM. Diagnosis of unintentional subdural anesthesia/analgesia: analyzing radiographically proven cases to define the clinical entity and to develop a diagnostic algorithm. Reg Anesth Pain Med 2009;34:12–6.
20. Abouleish E, Goldstein M. Migration of an extradural catheter into the subdural space. A case report. Br J Anaesth 1986;58:1194–7.
21. Elliott DW, Voyvodic F, Brownridge P. Sudden onset of subarachnoid block after subdural catheterization: a case of arachnoid rupture? Br J Anaesth 1996;76:322–4.
22. Orbegozo M, Sheikh T, Slogoff S. Subdural cannulation and local anesthetic injection as a complication of an intended epidural anesthetic. J Clin Anesth 1999;11:129–31.
23. Boezaart AP, Kadieva VS. Inadvertent extra-arachnoid (subdural) injection of a local anaesthetic agent during epidural anaesthesia. A case report. S Afr Med J 1992;81:325–6.

Challenges in Acute Pain Management

Kishor Gandhi, MD, MPH*, James W. Heitz, MD,
Eugene R. Viscusi, MD

KEYWORDS

• Acute pain • Challenging pain patient • Multimodal analgesia
• Analgesic gap

Adequate control of postoperative pain following surgery can be a challenging task.[1,2] Previous studies have shown that more than 50% of patients undergoing surgery report postoperative pain as a major concern, and that a majority of patients have unrelieved postoperative pain.[3] Uncontrolled pain in the postoperative period has been documented to result in several undesirable adverse events including myocardial ischemia and infarction, pulmonary infections, paralytic ileus, urinary retention, thromboembolism, impaired immune functions, and anxiety. In addition, poor pain control can lead to patient dissatisfaction, impaired patient rehabilitation, and prolonged hospitalization.[3] Patients who have well-controlled pain have an improved health-related quality of life, use fewer resources, reduce time lost from work, and have overall greater satisfaction with their experience.[4–8]

Although the benefits of pain control are uniformly recognized, hospitalized patients may not always benefit from optimal pain control because of the unique challenges some patients may present during the course of their hospitalization and surgery. Some difficulties in management can be attributed to patients who present with challenging clinical scenarios (ie, opioid-induced hyperalgesia, chronic pain patients with high tolerance to opioids, sickle cell disease, substance abuse, or metabolic or physical challenges that limit the dosing of pain medications). The clinician may also be unfamiliar with the management of medical problems that may increase the risk of opioid-induced side effects in patients with obstructive sleep apnea, the elderly, and the cognitively impaired. Patients with metabolic and neurologic disease states (such as renal failure, hepatic failure, and multiple sclerosis) have altered metabolism of drugs or unique risks for specific agents or techniques that may complicate the management of pain. Identifying an "ideal" analgesic that is free of undesired side effects and easy to administer may be difficult in such challenging clinical scenarios.[9]

Department of Anesthesiology, Jefferson Medical College, Thomas Jefferson University, 111 South 11th Street, Suite 8490, Philadelphia, PA 19107, USA
* Corresponding author.
E-mail address: Kishor.gandhi@jefferson.edu

Anesthesiology Clin 29 (2011) 291–309
doi:10.1016/j.anclin.2011.04.009
1932-2275/11/$ – see front matter © 2011 Elsevier Inc. All rights reserved.
anesthesiology.theclinics.com

ACUTE PAIN PROCESSING PATHWAYS

Pain is generated from local inflammation and nerve damage caused by trauma or temperature change (**Fig. 1**). Tissue trauma results in local release of inflammatory mediators such as bradykinins, 5-hydroxytryptamine, leukotrienes, prostaglandins (PGE_2, PGG_2, PGH_2), substance P, and histamine, which serve as activators of primary nociceptors. Receptors in the periphery detect changes of pain and temperature and transmit afferent signals in low-threshold myelinated Aβ fibers or high-threshold unmyelinated Aδ and C fibers. Signals reach the dorsal root ganglion via unmyelinated and myelinated noxious fibers and synapse in the dorsal horn of the spinal cord. The stimulus is then carried by second-order spinal neurons through

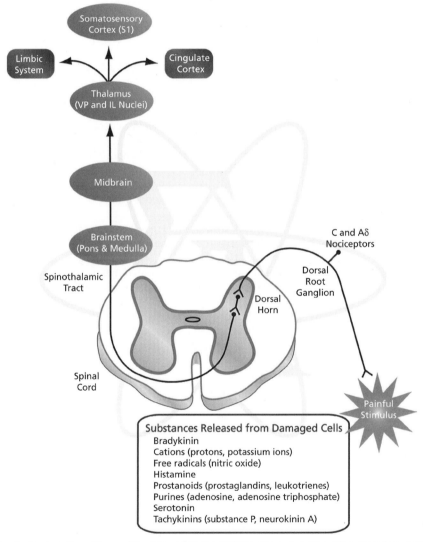

Fig. 1. Acute pain pathway. (*Courtesy of* Sigma-Aldrich, St Louis, MO; with permission. Available at: http://www.sigmaaldrich.com/life-science/cell-biology/learning-center/pathway-slides-and/ascending-pain-pathway.html.)

the neospinothalamic and paleospinothalamic tracts.[4] Modulation of pain transmission can occur at the level of the spinal cord dorsal horn or supraspinally at the brainstem and midbrain. Modulation involves a balance between excitatory effects of glutamine and the inhibitory effects of endogenous analgesics such as enkephalin (ENK), norepinephrine (NE), γ-aminobutyric acid (GABA), opioids, and α-adrenergics that target specific binding sites on 2-amino-3-(5-methyl-3-oxo-1,2-oxazol-4-yl) propanoic acid (AMPA), kainate, and N-methyl-D-aspartate (NMDA) receptors.[4] Once modified, noxious stimulus can transmit along axons from dorsal horn to thalamic cells and directly to the somatosensory cortex, which is involved in perception and localization of the stimulus.

OBJECTIVE PAIN ASSESSMENTS IN CHALLENGING PATIENTS

Because the pain experience has a subjective component, validated pain assessment tools are critical in appropriately assessing and treating pain. Because of the importance of pain treatment in the hospital setting, various organizations have created guidelines to assess and appropriately treat acute pain (World Health Organization, Agency for Healthcare Research and Quality, Joint Commission on Accreditation of Health Care Organizations [JCAHO]). The JCAHO has mandated treatment of pain as a basic human right.[10] JCAHO guidelines state that every patient has the right to assessment, treatment, and reassessment of pain.

Unidimensional pain intensity rating scales (Numeric Rating Scale [NRS], Verbal Descriptor Scale, Visual Analog Scale, Faces Pain Scale) can be used for patients who have an obvious cause of pain, but these metrics may not be adequate for more challenging patients (the elderly, and patients with visual/hearing impairment or cognitive impairments). A recent study measuring pain experiences in the elderly showed the NRS captured only part of the pain experience and should be supplemented by other forms of assessments.[11] Furthermore, unidimensional rating scales may not capture functional domains, and can contribute to misleading conclusions about treatment efficacy and recovery.[12] Multidimensional pain assessment tools such as Brief Pain Inventory, Initial Pain Assessment Inventory, and McGill Pain Questionnaire have been shown to be validated for complex pain seen in the perioperative period.[13] These measurement scales may better quantify pain and are reliable across various clinical settings.

PATIENT CHARACTERISTICS INFLUENCING MANAGEMENT
Opioid-Induced Hyperalgesia

Opioid-induced hyperalgesia (OIH) is a state in which patients being treated with opioids exhibit diminished pain threshold and enhanced sensitivity to pain. Despite dose escalation of opioids, patients may display reduced benefit from opioid therapy. OIH is considered a separate entity from analgesic tolerance; however, both may be present with dose escalation (**Fig. 2**). With OIH, escalating opioid treatment may paradoxically worsen the patient's pain perception.[14–16] It is difficult to distinguish clinically between tolerance and hyperalgesia.

OIH may result from hypersensitization of pronociceptive pathways in the peripheral or central nervous system (see **Fig. 1**).[17] While the mechanism of OIH is only beginning to be delineated, the process may be multifactorial, involving sensitization of primary and secondary afferents, enhanced release of neurotransmitters, and upregulation of spinal and supraspinal pathways. A critical component of OIH may be the activation of the excitatory NMDA receptor and the central glutamatergic system.[18] The link between NMDA receptors and the glutamatergic system has been shown by reversal

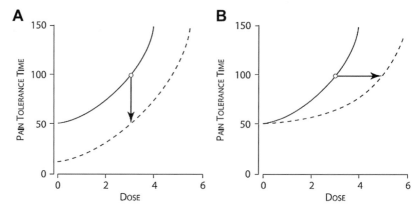

Fig. 2. Opioid dose-response relationship. (*A*) Opioid-induced hyperalgesia. (*B*) Opioid toler-ance in chronic pain patients. (*From* Chu LF, Angst MS, Clark D. Opioid-induced hyperalgesia in humans: molecular mechanism and clinical considerations. Clin J Pain 2008;24:480; with permission.)

of opioid-induced pain sensitivities via inhibition of both systems.[19] However, the glu-tamatergic system is likely involved in both tolerance and hyperalgesia. OIH has been demonstrated in patients receiving high-dose intraoperative opioids such as fentanyl and remifentanil.[20-22]

A proposed management strategy for OIH involves a multimodal analgesic approach targeting NMDA receptors, α2-agonists, and cyclooxygenase (COX)-2–specific inhibitors[17] (**Fig. 3**). Low-dose intraoperative and postoperative ketamine is an effective antagonist of NMDA receptors. Ketamine has been shown to reduce post-operative pain and opioid consumption. The NMDA receptor antagonism effects of ketamine may reduce postoperative opioid-induced hyperalgesia. Methadone, with its D-isomer acting as an NMDA receptor antagonist, may also reduce hyperalgesia. COX-2–specific inhibitors may attenuate the role of prostaglandin synthesis and NMDA receptor function in the central nervous system (CNS).[23-25] α2-Agonists such as clonidine have also been shown to reduce postoperative hyperalgesia when admin-istered intraoperatively. A multimodal approach is likely beneficial in the management of patients with presumed OIH.

Opioid Tolerance in Chronic Pain Patients

Tolerance (reduced analgesic effects of opioids) occurs in patients with prolonged opioid exposure. The development of tolerance with chronic opioid use results from desensitization of opioid antinociceptive pathways. Unlike opioid-induced hyperalge-sia, there is no change in baseline pain perception in opioid tolerance. Opioid toler-ance in chronic pain patients can usually be addressed by increasing opioid dose. Chronic opioid consumers may require a twofold to threefold increase in perioperative opioid dosing in comparison with opioid-naïve patients.[26] The molecular basis for opioid tolerance can be attributed to the desensitization of the μ-opioid receptor and second-messenger systems (protein kinase and G-protein) at the cellular level. Furthermore, activation of NMDA receptors and downregulation of glutamate trans-porter have been recently shown to take part in opioid tolerance.[19]

Appropriate management strategies of patients with opioid tolerance require iden-tification of these patients before surgery. Careful assessment of preoperative opioid requirements is vital. Perioperative management involves use of a multimodal drug

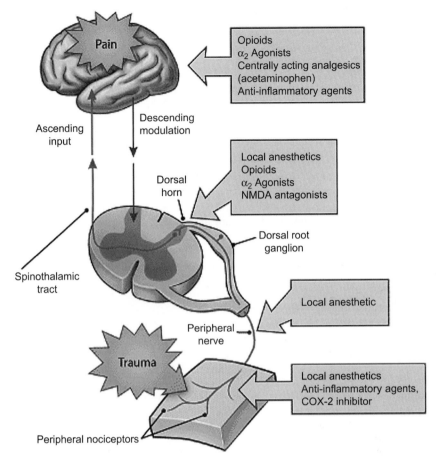

Fig. 3. Multimodal pain treatment. (*Modified from* Gottschalk A, Smith DS. New concepts in acute pain therapy: preemptive analgesia. Am Fam Physician 2001;63:1981; with permission.)

regimen.[27] Prior to surgery, patients may receive acetaminophen, celecoxib, gabapentin, or pregabalin. Both gabapentin and pregabalin act to inhibit $\alpha_2\delta$ subunit on the presynaptic voltage-gated calcium channel and attenuate the neuronal sensitization response. Perioperative use of pregabalin in addition to other nonopioid agents in total knee replacement has been shown to decrease opioid consumption and the incidence of neuropathic pain at 3 and 6 months after surgery.[28,29]

Intraoperative ketamine infusion (0.5 mg/kg bolus followed by 4 μg/kg/min infusion) and long-acting opioids for optimal comfort have demonstrated success. Ketamine, when given preoperatively and intraoperatively during spine surgery, was shown to reduce total morphine consumption and pain intensity for up to 6 weeks after surgery.[30] There were no differences in side effects when compared with placebo. Alternatively, intraoperative single bolus of methadone (0.2 mg/kg) has also shown a 50% reduction in postoperative opioid consumption and pain scores at 48 hours after surgery for complex spine procedures.[31]

Opioid-tolerant patients may see maximal benefits with regional anesthesia techniques using continuous neuraxial and peripheral nerve catheters for certain orthopedic and vascular procedures. Postoperative management will require supplemental opioid control of breakthrough pain as well as prevention of acute withdrawal from opioids, which best may be met with systemic opioids such as intravenous patient-controlled analgesia (PCA). However, it is helpful to maintain preoperative doses of extended-release opioids during the perioperative course. Postoperative ketamine infusion (up to 4 days) has also proved successful at the authors' institution in decreasing opioid requirements and improving analgesia in chronic pain patients with opioid tolerance.

Substance Abuse and Addiction

The National Survey on Drug Use and Health (NSDUH) estimates that more than 8% of the United States population older than 12 years in 2008 used illicit drugs in the previous month.[32] Patients with a history of opioid abuse and illicit drug addiction present a challenging scenario to the acute pain team. Patients with unrecognized chronic opioid exposure are at risk for opioid withdrawal and severe acute pain following surgery. Such patients may be dependent on polypharmacy through physician shopping or illicit street drugs. Commonly abused illicit drugs include marijuana, cocaine, 3,4-methylenedioxymethamphetamine (Ecstasy), and heroin.[32] Prescription opioid (eg, hydrocodone, oxycodone) abuse and misuse present a significant problem as well. It may be difficult to distinguish the addicted patient from the chronic pain patient or the addicted patient with chronic pain.[33,34] The patient with substance abuse will seek opioids despite effective pain control, while the chronic pain patient will titrate opioids to the degree of pain control. The addicted patient may not follow specific medication plans and may demand specific drugs for treatment, or claim allergies to nonopioids. The nonaddicted patient may display "drug-seeking" behavior if given inadequate doses (pseudoaddiction). Identification of the substance-abusing patient may be challenging and may not be revealed until the postoperative period when drug-seeking behavior is suspected.

Perioperative management of the known substance-abusing patient involves a carefully constructed plan during the preoperative, intraoperative, and postoperative course. The goal of treatment is to choose an appropriate strength of pain medication based on individual patient history.[35] A preoperative drug screen may be helpful to confirm whether the patient is actively using drugs and if so, which drugs are present. These patients should receive their long-acting opioids (methadone, extended-release oxycodone, extended-release morphine, and transdermal fentanyl) on the morning of the surgery to minimize acute opioid withdrawal in the perioperative period.[36] A preoperative dose of pregabalin, acetaminophen, and celecoxib will reduce sensitization of primary and secondary afferents.[17] Neuraxial and peripheral regional anesthesia techniques are recommended for orthopedic and vascular surgeries of upper and lower extremities. These techniques minimize pain and reduce the need for opioids during surgery.[37,38]

Intravenous PCA with morphine, hydromorphone, and fentanyl provide postsurgical analgesia before transition to oral agents alone. PCA has been studied extensively and has proved to be successful in opioid-dependent patients.[39,40] Minimizing postoperative opioid withdrawal is critical. A centrally acting α2-adrenergic agonist such as a clonidine transdermal (0.1–0.2 mg/h) patch is helpful in minimizing side effects and withdrawal in tolerant patients.[41] When appropriate, neuraxial and continuous peripheral nerve blocks can be continued with 0.2% ropivacaine or 0.1% bupivacaine up to 48 hours.[37,38] Opioid coadministration with local anesthetics to epidurals may improve analgesia and limit acute withdrawal symptoms. Continuation of a multimodal regimen including, acetaminophen, pregabalin, celecoxib, and ketorolac may provide pain relief for inflammatory and neuropathic components of pain.[17]

Sickle Cell Disease

Sickle cell disease is a genetically inherited disorder involving the β-globin chain production of red blood cells (RBCs). When an excess of defective RBCs are in the blood stream, patients develop painful crisis as a result of sickling of the RBCs in the microvasculature, followed by ischemia and activation of inflammatory pathways. Proinflammatory mediators released at the site of ischemia cause the release of vaso-constrictors, which exacerbate the vasoconstriction thus leading to worsening crisis. Local inflammation causes irritation of nerves, creating burning neuropathic-like pain. Crisis events are precipitated by physiologic stresses such as infections, dehydration, cold, or other external stressors. Patients with sickle cell syndrome typically display visceral or bone and joint pain during their "crisis" period, due to release of inflammatory mediators and stimulation of nociceptors.[42] It is common for these patients to display nociceptive as well as central and peripheral neuropathic pain. Often the anatomic location of the pain syndrome will vary by age and the extent of microinfarctions.[43] Differences in patient age and demographics can pose barriers in the reporting of pain during crisis events. Chronic pain syndromes as a result of sickle cell present later in life from avascular necrosis of long bones, leg ulcerations, and joints.[44]

Perioperative management of these patients involves careful planning to minimize any factors that can precipitate a painful crisis. Preparations include prewarming of operating rooms, adequate hydration of the patient before operation, and ample opioids to avoid a sickling event.[45] The first-line treatment for mild to moderate pain in sickle cell patients includes nonsteroidal anti-inflammatory drugs (NSAIDs), acetaminophen, celecoxib, and ketorolac.[43] Studies of patients treated with ketorolac infusion during vaso-occlusive crisis showed improved pain relief and reduced opioid requirements.[46] Tramadol, a synthetic central-acting analgesic, has also been shown to be effective in controlling mild to moderate sickle cell pain.[43] Meperidine is a poor opioid choice in sickle cell patients because of its short half-life (3 hours) and CNS stimulating activity of its metabolite (normeperidine).[47] Normeperidine has a half-life of 18 hours and can cause nervousness, tremors, and seizures. It is poorly excreted in sickle cell patients with kidney disease, leading to accumulation and increased the risk of seizures.

Because these patients often have significant opioid tolerance, they may benefit from PCA with appropriate (larger) patient control doses. Studies comparing opioids by intermittent versus PCA administration in sickle cell patients demonstrate greater satisfaction and pain relief in the PCA group.[48] Some clinicians may advocate the use of a basal infusion to avoid peaks and troughs of a bolus-only PCA program. However, PCA basal infusions should be used with caution because this has been associated with an increased risk of respiratory depression. A randomized trial comparing morphine PCA to a continuous infusion of morphine showed the PCA group to have decreased morphine consumption and reduced side effects.[49] The use of low-dose ketamine infusion has also been shown to reduce pain scores and opioid requirements during hospitalization.[50] Ketamine can be safely administered in low-dose infusion to decrease the amount of opioid consumption in this patient population.

Elderly and Cognitively Impaired Patients

The US Census Bureau estimates that 1 in 5 Americans (20.3%) will be 65 years or older by year 2030.[51] As "baby boomers" continue to age, increasing numbers of them will require hospitalizations and surgical care. As a consequence of normal physiologic changes of aging, the elderly present with pathophysiologic alterations such as decreased multisystem reserve, decreased cerebral and peripheral nervous system activity (cognitive impairment, delirium), and increased sensitivity to drugs (morphine, scopolamine, diphenhydramine, atropine). Delirium or cognitive impairment is a common postoperative complication seen in the elderly, and is often a worsening of underlying pathology that may have been unrecognized. It is estimated that up to 50% of the elderly population may suffer from postoperative delirium and cognitive dysfunction after orthopedic and cardiac surgeries.[52] The different classifications of cognitive impairment include dementia, mild cognitive impairment, postoperative cognitive dysfunction, delirium, postoperative delirium, and emergence delirium.[52] These cognitive impairments may continue up to 3 months after surgery in a minority of patients.

A careful management of perioperative technique is warranted in this high-risk population. Due to the altered pharmacodynamics of drugs, the elderly are more sensitive to anesthetics. General anesthesia will induce cognitive impairments as well as prolonged recovery times from anesthesia. Most opioids used for pain control have altered volume of distribution and decreased clearance, resulting in increased sensitivities.[53] Perioperative use of regional anesthesia has been shown to be effective in reducing morbidity (pneumonia, pulmonary embolism, myocardial infarction) and superior pain control.[7,54–56] Use of epidurals and peripheral nerve blocks has been shown to improve surgical outcome by decreasing opioid consumption, increasing ambulation and rehabilitative goals, and decreased length of hospital stay.[57] In addition, a multimodal approach with nonopioids such as NSAIDs, acetaminophen, ketorolac, and celecoxib can be used when there is a need to avoid the side-effect profile of opioids. Intravenous PCA may not be effective in patients who exhibit signs of dementia or delirium, due to inherent difficulties of operating the device.

Evaluations of mental status are rarely performed as part of routine preoperative assessments. Baseline deficits are often not recognized. Given the high incidence of perioperative changes of mental status in this age group, some preoperative assessment may be warranted to establish risk stratification and to better target anesthetic and analgesic techniques.

Sleep Apnea

Obstructive sleep apnea (OSA) is a syndrome in which the individual experiences recurrent complete or subtotal airway obstruction during sleep despite intact respiratory effort. The prevalence of OSA among adult Americans has been estimated at 2% of women and 4% of men.[58] However, there is increasing concern that the prevalence of OSA is rising with increasing obesity.

There is a considerable clinical overlap between OSA and central sleep apnea (CSA), and the conditions may present as a spectrum of disease. Individuals afflicted with sleep breathing disturbances may have both central and obstructive components.[59] Sleep apnea is defined as primarily OSA or CSA, depending on the relative proportion of obstructive versus central apneic episodes during a sleep study. In addition, some individuals with OSA develop treatment-emergent CSA after successful treatment. These observations have led to a more comprehensive concept of complex sleep apnea (CompSA). In a recent study of 1286 patients with primary OSA, 6.5% were noted to transiently develop treatment-emergent CSA after initiation of continuous positive airway pressure (CPAP) therapy, with 1% still affected at 8 weeks.[60]

It is important that clinicians maintain a high index of suspicion for OSA, because the majority of these individuals will be undiagnosed at the time they may need acute pain management. Although obesity is recognized as a marker of OSA, many patients with significant OSA are not obese. A history of loud snoring, daytime somnolence, witnessed apnea during sleep, and concurrent hypertension should alert the clinician to possible OSA.[61] It is estimated that 80% of males and 93% of females with moderate to severe OSA are undiagnosed.[62] Even among bariatric surgery patients, a very high risk group whose concurrent morbid obesity should raise clinical suspicion to possible OSA, the majority of cases of OSA are undiagnosed preoperatively.[63,64] This is unfortunate, because untreated OSA shortens life expectancy by more than 20 years and is linked to significant comorbidities including systemic hypertension, pulmonary hypertension, severe cardiovascular morbidity, and cardiac sudden death.[65–70] Recognition of sleep apnea has significant implications in the treatment of acute pain. Opioids, the most potent and widely used analgesics, can contribute to catastrophic respiratory events. An observed increase in the number of postoperative cardiopulmonary arrests by The Doctors Company in 2002 among patients receiving parenteral opioids later diagnosed with sleep apnea has raised concern about the safety of opioid analgesia in this population.[71]

The effects of opioids on the individual with sleep-disordered breathing have not been well studied. Hence, there is little evidence to guide therapy or craft guidelines. Opioids are known to inhibit the ventilatory response to both hypoxia and hypercapnia in healthy volunteers.[72] Opioids also cause obstructive apnea and hypoxia in the postoperative period in patients not identified with OSA.[73] Chronic opioid therapy with sustained-release opioids has been shown to increase the number of central and obstructive episodes of apnea, and is associated with sustained nocturnal hypoxia.[74] The respiratory depressant effects of opioids demonstrated in healthy individuals raise serious concerns for the consequences of opioids in patients with OSA, CSA, or CompSA.

In a study of volunteers with moderate OSA, opioid-induced apnea was observed during remifentanil infusion during sleep.[75] It is interesting that the number of episodes of obstructive apnea in these individuals decreased during opioid infusion, but this apparent "benefit" was more than offset by an increase in central apnea episodes. This apparent paradox is perhaps explained by the effect of opioids on rapid eye movement (REM) sleep. Opioids are known to decrease REM sleep. Pharyngeal muscle tone reaches a nadir during REM sleep, but REM sleep possibly offers protection against central apnea.[74,76] This finding is consistent with observations that CSA develops in up to 50% of patients on chronic opioid therapy.[77] Opioid-induced suppression of REM sleep is attenuated by prolonged use (REM rebound), so the effect of the remifentanil infusion on the number of obstructive episodes could not be predicted if the infusion had been continued beyond the short duration of the study.[78] Further studies clearly are needed to determine whether individuals with OSA will experience an increase in obstructive apnea as a late effect of opioid infusion, or if this finding can be replicated with other parenteral opioids in patients with sleep apnea.

Based on these findings, minimization of opioids and other sedatives in patients with known or suspected OSA, CSA, or CompSA is prudent. Route of opioid administration (intravenous, intramuscular, intrathecal, epidural) or administration technique (nurse-administered vs patient-controlled analgesia), does not affect the clinical risk.[79] Residual effect of anesthetics and sedatives may contribute to respiratory depression, but the sedating side effects of many adjuvant medications (antiemetics, antihistamines, β-blockers) should not be overlooked. Medications with mild sedating effects have the potential to cause serious adverse events when combined with opioids in patients with OSA.

In 2006, The American Society of Anesthesiologists Task Force of Perioperative Management of Patients with Obstructive Sleep Apnea released practice guidelines that included recommendations for postoperative pain management.[80] Although the task force did not make specific recommendations for analgesia in patients with OSA, they did recommend multimodal analgesic techniques to minimize opioids and to incorporate regional anesthesia and analgesia when possible. Epidural analgesia using only local anesthetics should be considered for postoperative analgesia. Nonpharmacological interventions, including ice and transcutaneous electrical stimulation, may be used when appropriate. The task force was equivocal on whether patient-controlled analgesia was preferable to nurse-controlled analgesia or whether patient-controlled analgesia with a basal infusion is safe. However, basal infusions with intravenous PCA are known to increase the risk of respiratory events.[81] Although CPAP has only been studied in non–perioperative settings, the task force recommended continuing CPAP postoperatively if not contraindicated for surgical reasons, but did not recommend institution of postoperative CPAP for patients not using it before surgery. Furthermore, the task force recommended that patients not be discharged home or to unmonitored settings until they were no longer at risk for postoperative respiratory depression. However, this raises the concern of how to predict when the patient is no longer at risk. While the guidelines clearly are helpful, clinical judgment is essential when guiding treatment decisions.

How best to monitor the sleep apnea patient requiring opioid therapy remains controversial. Although evidence is lacking, there is general agreement that continuous pulse oximetry is recommended for sleep apnea patients receiving opioids. Continuous pulse oximetry may not be available or difficult to manage at many institutions on general hospital floors, because the technology is prone to gaps and artifacts. Moreover, frequent alarms from repeated desaturations or artifacts may place a burden on nurses and be disruptive to the patient being monitored. Effective and accurate continuous pulse oximetry is best achieved in a monitored setting, but this approach considerably increases the cost of caring for these patients and consumes much-needed monitored bed resources. Capnography would also be effective as a monitor of respiration, and is becoming more widely available, but is still challenged by factors similar to pulse oximetry. Capnography may be a more sensitive and an earlier monitor of increasing respiratory difficulty. In a recent prospective cohort study at the Mayo Clinic, a combination of preoperative risk assessment combined with postanesthesia care unit observation for hypoxia was used to triage postoperative patients at risk for sleep apnea to the appropriate level of monitoring.[82] Further validation of this 2-phase screening for sleep apnea may allow for appropriate monitoring of high-risk individuals during opioid therapy for acute pain.

Beyond recommendations to limit opioid doses and general recommendations for monitoring, literature supporting greater safety of specific analgesic techniques or protocols is lacking. A prudent approach would follow the general principles of multimodal analgesia: use local anesthetic or regional anesthetic techniques whenever possible, preferably with a continuous (catheter) delivery, and supplement with nonopioid analgesics (acetaminophen, NSAIDs, or COX-2 inhibitors, antineuropathic pain agents, and ketamine).

OSA raises additional concerns in the ambulatory setting. While there are no hard and fast guidelines, prudence dictates caution. Patients with known severe OSA clearly should be approached with caution or even excluded from outpatient procedures. The use of nonopioids and nonsedating drugs with regional anesthetic and analgesic techniques becomes even more important. Careful and perhaps prolonged observation in the recovery unit may reveal obstructive episodes suggesting that admission for monitoring is indicated. With the increasing numbers of patients with OSA, the cost of excluding all of these patients from ambulatory surgery would be prohibitive. Many patients remain undiagnosed, complicating this scenario.

Although OSA may be obvious in many patients, the diagnosis remains unclear for many others. This fact, coupled with the lack of specific evidence for analgesic approaches or monitoring or the time period during which patients are at risk, makes for a challenging clinical scenario. For that matter, any patient receiving an opioid analgesic has some risk of respiratory depression. A simple, cost-effective, easy-to-use respiratory monitoring device is needed but remains elusive at this point.

Neurologic Disease

The patient with preexisting neurologic disease who may benefit from neuraxial or regional anesthesia in the treatment of acute pain offers a challenge to the clinician, prompting concerns that are simultaneously medical and medicolegal. Preexisting neurologic disease raises concern that patients may be particularly vulnerable to a second neurologic insult, the so-called double-crush phenomenon,[83] but also raises question of whether a clinician may be inappropriately assigned civil liability for a neurologic deficit that is merely coincidental. Multiple sclerosis, because of its often waxing and waning and unpredictable nature, presents a particularly vexing clinical conundrum.

Several older case reports have implicated spinal anesthesia and epidural anesthesia in contributing to exacerbations of multiple sclerosis.[84,85] More recently, anecdotal case reports have implicated peripheral nerve blocks in exacerbations as well.[86,87] However, anecdotal reports have also been cited as evidence of neuraxial anesthesia preventing exacerbations of multiple sclerosis after surgery.[88]

While there are no randomized controlled trials to guide therapy, several large retrospective studies have failed to show an increased risk of multiple sclerosis exacerbation after neuraxial anesthesia. In a retrospective review of vaginal deliveries at Brigham and Women's Hospital between 1982 and 1988, there was no significant difference in multiple sclerosis exacerbation between parturients receiving epidural anesthesia and those receiving local infiltration.[89] More recently, a review of 139 patients with multiple sclerosis receiving neuraxial anesthesia or analgesia at the Mayo Clinic between 1988 and 2000 did not reveal any exacerbations of the neurologic disease.[90]

While multiple sclerosis should not be considered an absolute contraindication to neuraxial or regional anesthesia, the clinician needs to carefully assess risk versus benefit on an individual basis. Whenever possible, informed consent should include a (documented) candid discussion with the patient about the risks and benefits of the proposed regional anesthetic, and acknowledgment that while the best evidence suggests that regional anesthesia can be used safely for patients with multiple sclerosis, there is no uniformity of opinion or certainty, as our knowledge of the risks is still evolving.[91]

Similar recommendations can be made for performance of regional anesthesia for rare demyelinating disorders such as Guillan-Barré syndrome (GBS) during the perioperative period. Published case reports have described worsening neurologic conditions after performance of epidural analgesia for labor and delivery.[92] However, neuraxial or regional anesthesia may be possible if the patient is treated effectively with intravenous immunoglobulin or plasmapheresis well in advance of surgery.[93] Although there are no published guidelines on the practice of regional anesthesia in GBS, the authors recommend caution in performance of nerve blocks because of the potential toxic effects of local anesthetic on unmyelinated nerves during the active phase of the illness.

Renal Disease

Acute pain management of the patient with end-stage renal disease (ESRD) presents an increasingly common challenge for the clinician. According the United States Renal Data System, at the conclusion of 2007 there were 526,343 ESRD patients in the United States; 341,264 on chronic hemodialysis, 26,340 on chronic ambulatory peritoneal dialysis, and 158,739 who had received renal transplants.[94] The number of individuals with chronic kidney disease (CKD) is significantly higher and is trending upward by as much as 10% each year, due to an aging population with an increasing incidence of diabetes mellitus and hypertension.[95] Pain is a common comorbidity in this patient population, and as many as one-third of patients with CKD are receiving opioids.[96] Safe use of analgesics in this population requires consideration not only for altered clearance of the parent drug but also altered clearance of metabolites, ability of parent drug and significant metabolites to be removed by hemodialysis in patients with ESRD, and for the potential for renal toxicity in patients with CKD or renal transplantation. Therefore, the clinician should understand not only the pharmacokinetics of the prescribed analgesic but the effect of CKD or hemodialysis on its pharmacokinetics.

Several commonly used opioids display favorable safety profiles with concurrent CKD or ESRD. Fentanyl elimination is greater than 99% hepatic, with transformation to primarily norfentanyl and to a lesser extent desproprionylfentanyl and hydroxyfentanyl.[97] Fentanyl has a long history of safe clinical use in patients with renal failure, as do the closely related alfentanil and sufentanil. This success is despite the fact that as molecules with large molecular weight and high protein binding, poor ability to dialyze these compounds from the blood would be expected. The metabolism of remifentanil is dissimilar, being metabolized by plasma cholinesterases, but it is also believed to be safe in renal failure patients. No increase in respiratory depression from remifentanil infusion was observed in patients with severe CKD.[98] Methadone has a favorable safety record in renal failure, despite having significant renal as well as hepatic elimination. Methadone and its metabolites cannot be dialyzed. However, there is evidence of complete excretion of the parent compound and its metabolites in feces in the setting of concurrent anuria.[99,100] Dose reduction of methadone is only necessary for severe CKD.[101]

Morphine, hydromorphone, and hydrocodone have been administered safely in renal failure patients, but need close monitoring for side effects and appropriate dose reduction because of the accumulation of active metabolites. Morphine undergoes hepatic metabolism, but its metabolites morphine-3-glucuronide, morphine-6-glucuronide, normorphine, and codeine all have renal elimination. Accumulation of morphine-6-glucuronide causes sedation. Although both morphine and morphine-6-glucuronide are effectively removed from the blood by hemodialysis, the slow diffusion of the latter out of the CNS makes elimination by hemodialysis clinically difficult. Hydrocodone is metabolized to hydromorphone by CYP2D6, and individuals lacking this enzyme experience no significant analgesia.[101] Hydromorphone is primarily metabolized to hydromorphine-3-glucuronide, whose accumulation in renal failure is associated with a neuroexcitatory phenomenon. Both hydrocodone and hydromorphone can be administered safely in patients with CKD but, like morphine, require appropriate dose reduction based on creatinine clearance.[100]

Several commonly prescribed analgesics are contraindicated in the presence of CKD. Meperidine, codeine, and propoxyphene are plagued by the accumulation of toxic metabolites causing unacceptable side-effect profiles.[100] Propoxyphene is particularly troublesome because it is poorly dialyzable and its metabolites are associated with respiratory depression, hypoglycemia, and cardiac conduction disturbances.[102,103] Aspirin and NSAIDs, although not associated with toxic metabolite accumulations, are relatively contraindicated for their ability to adversely affect the underlying CKD.

A unique clinical challenge arises from the need to provide analgesia to the ESRD patient not receiving hemodialysis, as may occur with end-of-life care. Such patients usually receive care via the incremental World Health Organization Analgesic Ladder approach.[104] Whereas Step 1, acetaminophen, may be administered safely in renal failure, there is no clear safe opioid for mild to moderate pain (Step 2). Tramadol may be the safest choice of the Step 2 opioids, but dose reduction is necessary. Good Step 3 opioid choices would include fentanyl or methadone.[105]

Hepatic Disease

The patient with hepatic insufficiency also provides a clinical challenge for analgesia. Unlike renal insufficiency, which can be quantitatively described by glomerular filtration rate or creatinine clearance allowing for dosing of opioids based on measured physiologic function, the severity of hepatic dysfunction is more difficult to measure precisely.

Because most opioids undergo hepatic metabolism, opioid dosing for the patient with hepatic dysfunction may be problematic. Unlike renal dysfunction, which typically results in accumulation of metabolites, hepatic dysfunction can cause accumulation of the parent drug or metabolites. As a general principle, oxidative processes are usually more severely affected than glucuronidation in patients with hepatic impairment.[106] However, the peak plasma concentration and elimination half-life of morphine, which undergoes primarily hepatic glucuronidation, have been demonstrated to be significantly elevated with patients with cirrhosis.[107] Acetaminophen is metabolized in part by glucuronidation. Hence, acetaminophen should be used with caution in the presence of hepatic impairment or known alcoholism.

All opioids must be administered cautiously. Long-acting and sustained-release opioids require extra caution. Codeine, which requires hepatic transformation to morphine for analgesia, should be avoided in severe hepatic dysfunction because its efficacy may be impaired.[108] Remifentanil, with its ultra-short half-life and its unique metabolism, has some attractive pharmacokinetic properties but its clinical utility for the treatment of acute pain is limited.

SUMMARY

The management of acute pain remains challenging, with many patients suffering inadequate pain control following surgery. Certain populations, as discussed in this review, are at unique risk for unrelieved pain. Evidence-based approaches taking into account specific needs and problems of patients will likely substantially improve their perioperative experience. To best serve these at-risk individuals, they must first be identified in the preoperative process. A plan can then be discussed with the patient and integrated into the anesthetic and analgesic strategy. A targeted multimodal approach to pain management should be considered the best clinical practice. Finally, the most challenging patients in acute pain may benefit most from the surveillance of an acute pain service that is able to monitor and coordinate care into the postoperative period.

REFERENCES

1. Apfelbaum JL, Chen C, Mehta SS, et al. Postoperative pain experience: results from a national survey suggest postoperative pain continues to be undermanaged. Anesth Analg 2003;97:534–40.
2. Warfield C, Kahn CH. Acute pain management: programs in U.S. hospitals and experiences and attitudes among U.S. adults. Anesthesiology 1995;83:1090–4.
3. Joshi GP, Ogunnaike BO. Consequences of inadequate postoperative pain relief and chronic persistent postoperative pain. Anesthesiol Clin North America 2005;23:21–36.
4. DeLeo JA. Basic science of pain. J Bone Joint Surg Am 2006;88(Suppl 2): 58–62.
5. Wall PD. The prevention of post operative pain. Pain 1988;32:289–90.
6. Chelly JE, Ben-David B, Williams BA, et al. Anesthesia and postoperative analgesia: outcomes following orthopedic surgery. Orthopedics 2003;26(8 Suppl): s865–71.
7. Rodgers A, Walker N, Schug S, et al. Reduction of postoperative mortality and morbidity with epidural or spinal anesthesia: results from overview of randomized trials. BMJ 2000;321:1493.
8. Munin M, Rudy T, Glynee N, et al. Early inpatient rehabilitation after elective hip and knee arthroplasty. JAMA 1998;279(11):847–52.
9. Heitz JW, Witkowski TA, Viscusi ER. New and emerging analgesic technologies for acute pain management. Curr Opin Anaesthesiol 2009;22:608–17.
10. Joint Commission on Accreditation of Health Care Organizations. Pain assessment and management, an organizational approach. Library of Congress Catalog No. 00-102701; 2000.
11. Wood BM, Nicholas MK, Blyth F, et al. Assessing pain in older people with persistent pain: the NRS is valid but only provides part of the picture. J Pain 2010;11(12):1259–66.
12. Hush JM, Refshauge KM, Sullivan G, et al. Do numerical rating scales and the Roland-Morris Disability Questionnaire capture changes that are meaningful to patients with persistent back pain? Clin Rehabil 2010;24:648–57.
13. Welchek CM, Matrangelo L, Sinatra RS, et al. Qualitative and quantitative assessment of pain. In: Sinatra RS, de Leon-Casasola OA, Ginsberg B, et al, editors. Acute pain management. New York: Cambridge University Press; 2009. p. 147–71.
14. Vadivelu N, Whitney CJ, Sinatra RS. Pain pathways and acute pain processing. In: Sinatra RS, de Leon-Casasola OA, Ginsberg B, et al, editors. Acute pain management. New York: Cambridge University Press; 2009. p. 3–20.
15. Ghori MK, Zang YF, Sinatra RS. Pathophysiology of acute pain. In: Sinatra RS, de Leon-Casasola OA, Ginsberg B, et al, editors. Acute pain management. New York: Cambridge University Press; 2009. p. 21–30.
16. Chu LF, Clark D, Angst MS. Molecular basis and clinical implications of opioid tolerance and opioid-induced hyperalgesia. In: Sinatra RS, de Leon-Casasola OA, Ginsberg B, et al, editors. Acute pain management. New York: Cambridge University Press; 2009. p. 114–43.
17. Chu LF, Angst MS, Clark D. Opioid-induced hyperalgesia in humans: molecular mechanism and clinical considerations. Clin J Pain 2008;24(6):479–96.
18. Mao J, Price DD, Mayer DJ. Thermal hyperalgesia in association with the development of morphine tolerance in rats: roles of excitatory amino acid receptors and protein kinase C. J Neurosci 1994;14:2301–12.

19. Truzillo KA, Akil H. Inhibition of morphine tolerance and dependence by the NMDA receptor antagonist MK-801. Science 1991;251:85–7.

20. Chi YY, Liu K, Wang JJ, et al. Intraoperative high dose fentanyl induces postoperative fentanyl tolerance. Can J Anaesth 1999;46:872–7.

21. Guignard B, Bossard AE, Coste C, et al. Acute opioid tolerance: intraoperative remifentanil increases postoperative pain and morphine requirement. Anesthesiology 2000;93:409–17.

22. Joly V, Richebe P, Guignard B, et al. Remifentanil-induced postoperative hyperalgesia and its prevention with small-dose ketamine. Anesthesiology 2005;103:147–55.

23. Malmberg AB, Yaksh TL. Hyperalgesia mediated by spinal glutamate or substance P receptor blocked by spinal cyclooxygenase inhibition. Science 1992;257:1276–9.

24. Yaksh TL, Malmberg AB. Spinal actions of NSAIDs in blocking spinally medicated hyperalgesia: the role of cyclooxygenase products. Agents Actions Suppl 1993;41:89–100.

25. Powell KJ, Hosokawa A, Bell A, et al. Comparative effects of cyclooxygenase and nitric oxide synthase inhibition on the development and reversal of spinal opioid tolerance. Br J Pharmacol 1999;127:631–44.

26. De Leon-Casasola OA, Myers DP, Donaparthe S, et al. A comparison of postoperative epidural analgesia between patients with chronic cancer taking high dose of oral opioids versus opioid-naïve patients. Anesth Analg 1993;76:302–7.

27. Carroll IR, Angst MS, Clark JD. Management of perioperative pain in patients chronically consuming opioids. Reg Anesth Pain Med 2004;29:574–91.

28. Clarke H, Pereira S, Kennedy D, et al. Gabapentin decreases morphine consumption and improves functional recovery following total knee arthroplasty. Pain Res Manag 2009;14:217–22.

29. Buvanendran A, Kroin JS, Della Valle CJ, et al. Perioperative oral pregabalin reduces chronic pain after total knee arthroplasty: a prospective, randomized controlled trial. Anesth Analg 2010;110:199–207.

30. Loftus RW, Yeager MP, Clark JA, et al. Intraoperative ketamine reduces perioperative opiate consumption in opiate-dependent patients with chronic back pain undergoing back surgery. Anesthesiology 2010;113:639–46.

31. Gottschalk A, Durieux ME, Nemergut EC. Intraoperative methadone improves postoperative pain control in patients undergoing complex spine surgery. Anesth Analg 2010;112(1):218–23.

32. US Department of Health and Human Services. Office of Applied Statistics, Substance Abuse and Mental Health Services Administration (SAMHSA). Drug Abuse Warning Network (DAWN). The DAWN Report: Opiate-related drug misuse deaths in six states: 2003. Rockville (MD): SAMHSA; 2006. Issue.

33. Mitra S, Sinatra RS. Patients with opioid dependence and substance abuse. In: Sinatra RS, de Leon-Casasola OA, Ginsberg B, et al, editors. Acute pain management. New York: Cambridge University Press; 2009. p. 564–80.

34. Mitra S, Sinatra RS. Perioperative management of acute pain in the opioid-dependent patient. Anesthesiology 2004;101:212–27.

35. Prater CD, Zylstra RG, Miller KE. Successful pain management for the recovering addicted patient. J Clin Psychiatry 2002;4:125–31.

36. Mehta V, Langford RM. Acute pain management for opioid dependent patient. Anaesthesia 2006;61:269–76.

37. Liu S, Carpenter RL, Neal JM. Epidural anesthesia and analgesia. Their role in postoperative outcome. Anesthesiology 1995;82:474–506.

38. Schug SA, Fry RA. Continuous regional analgesia in comparison with intravenous opioid administration for routine postoperative pain control. Anaesthesia 1994;49:528–32.
39. Savage SR. Principles of pain treatment in the addicted patient. In: Graham AW, Schultz TK, editors. Principles of addiction medicine. 2nd edition. Chevy Chase (MD): American Society of Addiction Medicine, Inc; 1998. p. 919–44.
40. Locolano CF. Perioperative pain management in the chemically dependent patient. J Perianesth Nurs 2000;15:329–47.
41. Lobmaier P, Gossop M, Waal H, et al. The pharmacological treatment of opioid addiction—a clinical perspective. Eur J Clin Pharmacol 2010;66:537–45.
42. Varadarajan JL, Weisman SJ. Acute pain management in sickle cell disease patients. In: Sinatra RS, de Leon-Casasola OA, Ginsberg B, et al, editors. Acute pain management. New York: Cambridge University Press; 2009. p. 550–63.
43. Ballas SK. Current issues in sickle cell pain and its management. Hematology Am Soc Hematol Educ Program 2007;97–105.
44. McClish DK, Smith WR, Dahman BA, et al. Pain site frequency and location in sickle cell disease: the PiSCES project. Pain 2009;145:246–51.
45. Okomo U, Meremikwu. Fluid replacement therapy for acute episodes of pain in people with sickle cell disease. Cochrane Database Syst Rev 2007;2:CD005406.
46. Perli E, Finke H, Castro O, et al. Enhancement of pain control with ketorolac tromethamine in patients with sickle cell vaso-occlusive crisis. Am J Hematol 1994;46:43–7.
47. Hagmeyer KO, Mauro LS, Mauro VF. Meperidine-related seizures associated with patient-controlled analgesia pumps. Ann Pharmacother 1993;27:29–32.
48. Gonzales ER, Bahal N, Hansen LA, et al. Intermittent injection vs. patient-controlled analgesia for sickle cell crisis pain. Comparison in patients in the emergency department. Arch Intern Med 1991;151:1371–8.
49. Van Beers EJ, van Tuijn CFJ, Nieuwkerk PT, et al. Patient-controlled analgesia versus continuous infusion of morphine during vaso-occlusive crisis in sickle cell disease, a randomized controlled trial. Am J Hematol 2007;82:955–60.
50. Zempsky WT, Loisella KA, Corsi JM, et al. Use of low-dose ketamine infusion for pediatric patients with sickle cell disease-related pain: a case series. Clin J Pain 2010;26:163–7.
51. US Bureau of the Census. An aging world: 2001. Available at: http://www.census.gov/prod/2001pubs/p95-01-1.pdf. Accessed August 10, 2010.
52. Halazynski TM, Saidi N, Lopez J. Acute pain management for elderly high-risk and cognitively impaired patients: rationale for regional analgesia. In: Sinatra RS, de Leon-Casasola OA, Ginsberg B, et al, editors. Acute pain management. New York: Cambridge University Press; 2009. p. 514–36.
53. Shafer SL. The pharmacology of anesthetic drugs in elderly patients. Anesthesiol Clin North America 2000;18:1–29.
54. Ballantyne JC, Carr DB, deFerranti S, et al. The comparative effects of postoperative analgesic therapies on pulmonary outcome: cumulative meta- analyses of randomized, controlled trials. Anesth Analg 1998;86:598–612.
55. Wu CL, Hurley RW, Anderson GF. Effects of postoperative epidural analgesia on morbidity and mortality following surgery in Medicare patients. Reg Anesth Pain Med 2004;29:525–33.
56. Liu SS, Block BM, Wu CL. Effects of perioperative central neuraxial analgesia on outcome after coronary artery bypass surgery: a meta-analysis. Anesthesiology 2004;101:153–61.

57. Kehlet H. Multimodal approach to control postoperative pathophysiology and rehabilitation. Br J Anaesth 1997;78:606–27.
58. Young T, Palta M, Dempsey J, et al. The occurrence of sleep disordered breathing among middle aged adults. N Engl J Med 1993;328:1230–5.
59. Badr MS, Toiber F, Skatrud JB, et al. Pharyngeal narrowing/occlusion during central sleep apnea. J Appl Physiol 1995;78:1806–15.
60. Javaheri S, Smith J, Chung E. The prevalence and natural history of complex sleep apnea. J Clin Sleep Med 2009;5:205–11.
61. Chung F, Yegneswaran B, Liao P, et al. STOP questionnaire: a tool to screen patients for obstructive sleep apnea. Anesthesiology 2008;108:812–21.
62. Young T, Evans L, Finn L, et al. Estimation of clinically diagnosed proportion of sleep apnea syndrome in middle-aged men and women. Sleep 1997;20:705–6.
63. Frey WC, Pilcher J. Obstructive sleep-related breathing disorders in patients evaluated for bariatric surgery. Obes Surg 2003;13:676–83.
64. O'Keefe T, Patterson EJ. Evidence supporting routine polysomnography before bariatric surgery. Obes Surg 2004;14:23–6.
65. Young T, Finn L. Epidemiological insights into public health burden of sleep disordered breathing: sex differences in survival among sleep clinic patients. Thorax 1998;53(Suppl 3):S16–9.
66. Peppard PE, Young T, Palta M, et al. Prospective study of the association between sleep-disordered breathing and hypertension. N Engl J Med 2000;342:1378–84.
67. Krieger J, Sforza E, Apprill M, et al. Pulmonary hypertension, hypoxemia, and hypercapnia in obstructive sleep apnea patients. Chest 1989;96:729–37.
68. Martin JM, Carrizo SJ, Vicente E, et al. Long term cardiovascular outcomes in men with obstructive sleep apnoea-hypopnoea with or without treatment with continuous positive airway pressure: an observation study. Lancet 2005;365:1046–53.
69. Yaggi HK, Concato J, Kernan WN, et al. Obstructive sleep apnea as a risk factor for stroke and death. N Engl J Med 2005;353:2034–41.
70. Gami AS, Howard DE, Olson EJ, et al. Day-night pattern of sudden death in obstructive sleep apnea. N Engl J Med 2005;352:1206–14.
71. Lofsky A. Sleep apnea and narcotic postoperative pain medicine. A morbidity and mortality risk. Anesthesia Patient Safety Foundation Newsletter 2002;17:24–5.
72. Weil JV, McCullough RE, Kline JS, et al. Diminished ventilatory response to hypoxia and hypercapnia after morphine in normal man. N Engl J Med 1975;292:1103–6.
73. Catley DM, Thornton C, Jordan C, et al. Pronounced episodic oxygen desaturation in the postoperative period: its association with ventilator pattern and analgesic regimen. Anesthesiology 1985;63:20–8.
74. Farney RJ, Walker JM, Cloward TV, et al. Sleep-disordered breathing associated with long-term opioid therapy. Chest 2003;123:632–9.
75. Bernards CM, Knowlton SL, Schmidt DF, et al. Respiratory and sleep effects of remifentanil in volunteers with moderate obstructive sleep apnea. Anesthesiology 2009;110:41–9.
76. Horner RL. Respiratory motor activity: influence of neuromodulars and implications for sleep disordered breathing. Can J Physiol Pharmacol 2007;85:155–65.
77. Eckert DJ, Jordan AS, Merchia P, et al. Central sleep apnea: pathophysiology and treatment. Chest 2007;131:595–607.

78. Endo T, Roth C, Landolt HP, et al. Selective REM sleep deprivation in humans. Effects on sleep and EEG. Am J Physiol 1998;274:R1186–94.

79. Isono S. Obstructive sleep apnea of obese adults: pathophysiology and perioperative airway management. Anesthesiology 2009;110:908–21.

80. ASA Task Force on Perioperative Management of Patients with Obstructive Sleep Apnea. Practice guidelines for the perioperative management of patients with obstructive sleep apnea. Anesthesiology 2006;104:1081–93.

81. Parker RK, Holtmann B, White PF. Patient-controlled analgesia. Does a concurrent opioid infusion improve pain management after surgery? JAMA 1991; 266(14):1947–52.

82. Gali B, Whalen FX, Schroeder DR, et al. Identification of patients at risk for postoperative respiratory complications using a preoperative obstructive sleep apnea screening tool and postanesthesia care assessment. Anesthesiology 2009;110:869–77.

83. Upton AR, McComas AJ. The double crush in nerve entrapment syndromes. Lancet 1973;2:359–62.

84. Fleiss AN. Multiple sclerosis appearing after spinal anesthesia. Anesthesiology 1950;11:381–2.

85. Warren TM, Datta S, Ostheimer GW. Lumbar epidural anesthesia in a patient with multiple sclerosis. Anesth Analg 1982;61:1022–3.

86. Koff MD, Cohen JA, McIntyre JJ, et al. Severe brachial plexopathy after ultrasound-guided single-injection nerve block for total shoulder arthroplasty in a patient with multiple sclerosis. Anesthesiology 2008;108:325–8.

87. Kocer B, Ergan S, Nazliel B. Isolated abducens nerve palsy following mandibular block articaine anesthesia, a first manifestation of multiple sclerosis: a case report. Quintessence Int 2009;40:251–6.

88. Okada A, Hirose M, Shimizu K, et al. Perioperative anesthetic management of a patient with multiple sclerosis. Masui 2009;58:772–4.

89. Bader AM, Hunt CO, Datta S, et al. Anesthesia for the obstetric patient with multiple sclerosis. J Clin Anesth 1988;1:21–4.

90. Hebl JR, Horlocker TT, Schroeder DR. Neuraxial anesthesia and analgesia in patients with preexisting central nervous system disorders. Anesth Analg 2006;103:223–8.

91. Drake E, Drake M, Bird J, et al. Obstetric regional blocks for women with multiple sclerosis: a survey of UK experience. Int J Obstet Anesth 2006;15: 115–23.

92. Wiertlewski S, Armelle M, Sophie D, et al. Worsening of neurologic symptoms after epidural anesthesia for labor in a Guillain-Barre Patient. Anesth Analg 2004;98:825–7.

93. Kocabas S, Karaman S, Firat V, et al. Anaesthetic management of Guillain-Barre syndrome in pregnancy. J Clin Anesth 2007;19:299–302.

94. The United States Renal Data Systems (USRDS). Available at: http://www.usrds.org/2009/fb/2009_booklet/booklet.html. Accessed August 4, 2010.

95. Coresh J, Selvin E, Stevens LA. Prevalence of chronic kidney disease in the United States. JAMA 2007;298:2038–47.

96. Davison SN. Pain in hemodialysis patients: prevalence, cause, severity, and management. Am J Kidney Dis 2003;42:1239–47.

97. Labroo RB, Paine MF, Thummel KE, et al. Fentanyl metabolism by human hepatic and intestinal cytochrome P450 3A4: implications for interindividual variability in disposition, efficacy and drug interactions. Drug Metab Dispos 1997;25:1072–80.

98. Hoke JF, Shlugman D, Dershwitz M, et al. Pharmacokinetics and pharmacody-namics of remifentanil infusion in persons with renal failure compared with healthy volunteers. Anesthesiology 1997;87:533.
99. Kreek MJ, Schecter AJ, Gutjahr CL, et al. Methadone use in patients with chronic renal disease. Drug Alcohol Depend 1980;5:197–205.
100. Dean M. Opioids in renal failure and dialysis patients. J Pain Symptom Manage 2004;28:497–504.
101. Lurcott G. The effects of the genetic absence and inhibition of CYP2D6 on the metabolism of codeine and its derivatives, hydrocodone and oxycodone. Anesth Prog 1998;45:154–6.
102. Mauer SJ, Paxon CL, von Hartizsch B, et al. Hemodialysis in an infant with propoxyphene intoxication. Clin Pharmacol Ther 1975;17:88–92.
103. Barkin RL, Barkin SJ, Barkin DS. Propoxyphene (dextropropoxyphene): a critical review of a weak opioid analgesic that should remain in antiquity. Am J Ther 2006;13:534–42.
104. World Health Organization. Available at: http://www.who.int/cancer/palliative/painladder/en/. Accessed August 4, 2010.
105. Murtagh FEM, Chai M, Donohoe P, et al. The use of opioid analgesia in end-stage renal disease in patients managed without dialysis: recommenda-tions or practice. J Pain Palliat Care Pharmacother 2007;21:5–16.
106. Congiu M, Mashford ML, Slavin JL, et al. UDP glucuronosyltransferase. Drug Metab Dispos 2002;30:129–34.
107. Hasselstrom J, Eriksson S, Persson A, et al. The metabolism and bioavailability of morphine in patients with severe liver cirrhosis. Br J Clin Pharmacol 1990;29:289–97.
108. Gasche Y, Daali Y, Fathi M, et al. Codeine intoxication associated with ultralipid CYP2D6 metabolism. N Engl J Med 2004;351:2827–33.

New Concepts in Acute Pain Management: Strategies to Prevent Chronic Postsurgical Pain, Opioid-Induced Hyperalgesia, and Outcome Measures

Irina Grosu, MD, Marc de Kock, MD, PhD*

KEYWORDS

• Hyperalgesia • Chronic postsurgical pain • Pain • Anesthesia

Chronic postsurgical pain (CPSP) is a pain syndrome that has attracted attention for more than 10 years. The criteria for this diagnostic entity were established by the International Association for the Study of Pain (IASP) in 1999. CPSP is a pain syndrome that develops postoperatively and lasts for at least 2 months in the absence of other causes for pain (eg, recurrence of malignancy, chronic infection, and so forth). Pain continuing from a preexisting disease is not considered as CPSP.[1] In this article, the authors discuss the etiopathogenesis of CPSP and interventions that can help prevent and treat this condition.

The following case report illustrates the particular clinical presentation of CPSP.

A 48-year-old active businesswoman was scheduled for a Nissen fundoplication by an open thoracic (Belsey) approach. This surgical intervention was indicated because of acid reflux symptoms resistant to antireflux medications. The type of surgery was chosen based on the demonstration of a Barrett esophagus by the radiological examination. The patient was obese with a body mass index (BMI; calculated as the weight in kilograms divided by the height in meters squared)

The authors have no conflict of interest.
Department of Anesthesia and Perioperative Medicine, Catholic University of Louvain, St Luc Hospital, 10 Avenue Hippocrate, 1200 Brussels, Belgium
* Corresponding author.
E-mail address: dekock@anes.ucl.ac.be

Anesthesiology Clin 29 (2011) 311–327
doi:10.1016/j.anclin.2011.04.001   anesthesiology.theclinics.com
1932-2275/11/$ – see front matter © 2011 Elsevier Inc. All rights reserved.

of 30 and had quit smoking 10 years prior to surgery and thus was documented to be of the American Society of Anesthesiologists physical status 2. The procedure was done under general anesthesia combined with a thoracic epidural analgesia. Postoperative pain was managed using patient-controlled thoracic epidural analgesia (PCEA) with a bupivacaine-sufentanil mixture and intravenous proparacetamol until the fifth postoperative day. During the following days, proparacetamol and tramadol replaced the PCEA. The postoperative course was uneventful. The patient was discharged home on the eleventh postoperative day.

Six months later, this patient was readmitted for a partial costal resection for unbearable right thoracic pain at the old thoracotomy site. This procedure was ineffective to relieve the pain, and the patient was thus referred to the pain clinic. Multiple attempts with escalating analgesic medications and local infiltrations were performed with only modest results. The patient finally benefited from a spinal cord stimulator but could not return to work because of pain.

During the initial 6 months after her thoracotomy, the patient consulted the surgeon 3 times and the general practitioner more than 10 times, who referred her to 2 different neurologists and 1 psychiatrist. However, the patient never consulted an anesthetist or a chronic pain physician!

A few important lessons can be drawn form this case report.

In most cases of CPSP, the primary anesthetist providing the initial anesthesia to the patient is not aware of the occurrence of CPSP because this syndrome develops when the patient is already back home.

Further, in some patients, CPSP diminishes or resolves over time, whereas for some (0.5%–1.5% of all the patients undergoing surgery) it becomes an invalidating chronic pain necessitating frequent visits to chronic pain facilities.[2] Therefore, prevention is of critical importance.

Before discussing the strategies to prevent CPSP, some facts about CPSP are mentioned.

WHAT IS THE INCIDENCE OF CPSP

CPSP occurs in 10% to 50% of individuals after common operations, such as groin hernia repair, breast and thoracic surgery, leg amputation, orthopedic procedures (donor site pain, complex regional pain syndrome), and coronary artery bypass surgery (**Box 1**).[3] More worrisome, however, is the fact that 2% to 10% of these patients evolve toward developing severe chronic pain. The high number of patients undergoing surgery per year makes CPSP a potentially significant problem of public health. This fact, however, deserves several comments.

The data supporting the incidence of CPSP are estimations extrapolated mostly from retrospective evaluations.[3] In these series, it is not easy to make a clear-cut distinction between preexisting and postoperative persisting pains. Patients, questioned postoperatively, often do not accurately remember if the pain was present before or after surgery and for how long the pain had lasted. Consequently, an overvaluation of the real incidence of the phenomenon cannot be totally ruled out. Moreover, in the few prospective studies available in the literature (most including a small number of patients), the incidence of CPSP is lower than that reported in the retrospective ones.[4–6] For this reason, there is clearly a need for large prospective evaluations based on the exact definition of CPSP according to the IASP.[1]

Nevertheless, even if the exact incidence of CPSP is unknown, this problem is of critical importance when considering surveys of patients consulting chronic pain facilities. These facilities reveal that for a large fraction of patients (30% according to Crombie and colleagues[7]), the start of the pain syndrome was consecutive to surgery.

Box 1
Incidence of CPSP after various interventions

- Limb amputation: 60%–80%

- Total hip arthroplasty: 30%

- Hysterectomy: 5%–30%

- Caesarean section: 10%

- Breast surgery 20%–50%

- Groin hernia surgery: 10%

- Sternotomy: 20%

- Thoracotomy: 25%–60%

Data from Perkins FM, Kelhet H. Chronic pain as an outcome from surgery. A review of predictive factors. Anesthesiology 2000;93:1123–33.

This high incidence of CPSP is probably not a real surprise. The high incidence may be related to the ever-increasing incidence of diseases associated with proinflammatory states, such as asthma, inflammatory bowel diseases, or fibromyalgia, in developed countries. Asthma for example was rare in 1900. At present, asthma affects 15 million people in the United States.[8] One explanation could be that the population evolves toward a greater vulnerability to proinflammatory processes, and CPSP is just one of these processes. Moreover, an ever-increasing part of the population is obese, and obesity is recognized as a proinflammatory condition.[9] Obesity is also recognized as a favoring factor for the development of CPSP (see later).

CPSP is a pain syndrome that potentially affects a large and probably an increasing number of surgical patients. CPSP occurs after not only extensive but also simple procedures. In patients with chronic pain, a history of surgery is frequently noted as the starting point of the pain problem. Large prospective studies are, however, mandatory to determine the exact incidence of CPSP and to isolate the epidemiologic predisposing factors. These large series should also include a reproducible quantification of the physical functioning and emotional well-being of the patients.

MECHANISMS UNDERLYING THE DEVELOPMENT OF CPSP

CPSP syndrome results probably from a dysfunction of the mechanisms underlying secondary hyperalgesia.[10] At present, the cause of this dysfunction is not known. It is clear that long-lasting noxious stimulations, inflammation, or damages to the neuronal tissues, which all occur to some extent after surgery, give rise to a neuronal hyperexcitability that is mostly relatively short lasting and associated with reversible plastic changes in neuronal connectivity. In some circumstances, such as intense noxious stimulation, proinflammatory context, vulnerable patients, as well as persistent and more profound changes in transmitters, receptors, and ion channels, neuronal connectivity occurs, leading to irreversible plastic changes and CPSP. However, why some patients develop CPSP and others do not is still an unresolved question.

Pain has an important physiologic role, being a sensory modality that normally serves an adaptive function. Pain is a sensory warning system that activates protective reflexes and determines brain adaptive behaviors. Pain, as any sensory modality, implicates both perception (something happens) and discrimination (what is happening now is different of the previous perception). Distinct physiologic mechanisms underlie these 2 functions. There are specific pain receptors (the nociceptors), and their perception can be significantly reduced (descending inhibitory controls) or amplified (primary and secondary hyperalgesia) at peripheral and central levels. This capacity to modulate pain perception is, in fact, the physiologic basis for discrimination. Unlike other sensory modalities, pain perception is strongly linked to the immune system (inflammatory reaction consecutive to tissue destruction). Pain can be powerfully amplified by activation of peripheral immune cells associated with peripheral nerves and by the activation of immunelike glial cells (microglia and astrocytes) within the central nervous system.[11]

Postoperative pain is a particular type of pain. This pain is definitively not to be considered as a simple symptom that disappears with wound healing or even as a symptom consecutive to an accidental trauma. Although most patients expect to experience pain after surgery, the pain in this setting can be exaggerated by psychological and pharmacologic factors. For example, the level of anxiety is known to correlate with the severity of pain from nociceptive stimuli. In addition, surgical tissue injury occurs during anesthesia, which may be important because anesthetic drugs interfere with sensory perception, but the effects of these drugs on pain processing are not necessarily unidirectional. For example, potent opioids produce both antinociception and hyperalgesia.[12] Halogenated vapors given to produce unconsciousness and amnesia also activate peripheral pronociceptive ionic channels, thereby augmenting neurogenic inflammation.[13]

Surgical trauma is associated with hyperalgesia (exacerbated pain in response to noxious stimulation) and allodynia (pain perceived to normally nonnoxious stimuli). Trauma leads to the release of inflammatory mediators at the site of injury, resulting in a reduction of pain threshold at the site of injury (primary hyperalgesia) and in the surrounding uninjured tissue (secondary hyperalgesia). Secondary hyperalgesia is the distinguishing mark of central sensitization, which is an activity-dependent increase in the excitability of spinal neurons (windup) as a result of persistent exposure to afferent input from peripheral neurons and inflammatory mediators. Prolonged central sensitization has the capacity to lead to permanent alterations in the central nervous system, including the disappearance of inhibitory interneurons, replacement with new afferent excitatory neurons, and establishment of new excitatory connections.[14] Central sensitization is not an abnormal but a modified perceptual response to a normal sensory input and results in the spread of sensitivity well beyond the peripheral site of injury (secondary hyperalgesia). Central sensitization is a modification of the homeostasis, leading to a new state necessary for healing. For example, hyperalgesia surrounding the wounded area promotes behavioral adaptation required for survival. It is also of critical importance to oppose the hypoalgesic influences induced by the trauma itself (stress induced or autoanalgesia). Hyperalgesia is part of the mechanism enabling discrimination in pain perception.

In the context of CPSP, secondary hyperalgesia has prompted attention for several reasons.

First, secondary hyperalgesia reflects transformations within the central nervous system, which share many features of mechanisms of memory. Both are dependent on the excitatory neurotransmission (glutaminergic neurotransmission). This particular type of transmission through the medium of N-methyl-D-aspartate (NMDA) receptors is involved in long-term modification of neuronal connectivity (neuroplasticity) and is demonstrated to play a key role in the induction and maintenance of central sensitization during physiologic and pathologic pain states.[15]

Second, secondary hyperalgesia is exemplary of the neuroimmune interactions in pain perception. Traumatic surgical injury to the peripheral nerve produces changes at the site of injury as well as in the dorsal root ganglia and dorsal horn of the spinal cord. Changes in dorsal horn involve neuronal and nonneuronal cells, begin within hours, and persist for up to months after surgery. Of particular interest are the changes involving nonneuronal tissues, such as the microglia (the resident macrophages of the brain and spinal cord). Recently, specific neuron-microglia-neuron signaling pathways have been elucidated. Microglia in the dorsal horn suppress neuronal inhibition by a sequence of steps (brain-derived neurotrophic factors), leading to an increase in intracellular chloride concentration in dorsal horn nociceptive output. Products released by activated microglia, including cytokines such as interleukin (IL)-1β, IL-6, and tumor necrosis factor α, are normally expressed in low concentrations in the spinal cord; however, this expression increases after peripheral nerve injury and peripheral inflammation.

These neuronal/immune interactions account for the symptoms of neuropathic pain associated with CPSP.[11] Dysfunctions of these mechanisms are suspected to induce a prolonged state of sensitization clinically manifested by CPSP.[10,16]

Clinically, patients developing CPSP presented a larger area of secondary hyperalgesia surrounding the surgical wound measured by the von Frey hairs than those not presenting with CPSP.[6,17–19]

The problem remains as to how and why physiologic posttraumatic hyperalgesia develop in pathologic hyperalgesia. One explanation could be the extent of surgery-associated neuronal damages. Nerve injury leads to abnormal plasticity resulting in ectopic pacemakerlike activity and nonphysiologic central sensitization. Nerve injury produces long-lasting central changes by potent immune tissue activation. This hypothesis is sustained by the fact that most of the time, the characteristics of CPSP are those of neuropathic pain.[20] Nevertheless, not all patients presenting with nerve damage consecutive to surgery develop CPSP,[21] and CPSP does not always or exclusively match the characteristics of neuropathic pain.[22]

Another explanation could be found in the preoperative antiinflammatory/proinflammatory status of the patient. In some patients, the proinflammatory response might be particularly intense or inadequate in regard to the surgical trauma. Arguments for this hypothesis exist. In developed countries, the incidence of obesity, which is a proinflammatory disease, is still increasing,[9] and CPSP occurs more frequently in obese patients. Moreover, in patients developing CPSP, a history of inflammatory process in the part of the body concerned by surgery is often noted.[18] This concept supports a kind of algesic proinflammatory priming favoring the development of the syndrome.[22]

Another circumstance related to the patient may also account for the development of CPSP. As previously noted, hyperalgesia is a physiologic process implicated in discrimination. Recently, a deregulation of the discrimination process was incriminated in the occurrence of some pathologies, such as fibromyalgia, in which patients show robust perceptual amplification of all the sensory modalities, including pain perception (the hypervigilance theory).[23] Patients with fibromyalgia share many common characteristics with those at risk of developing important acute postoperative pain and CPSP (female gender, anxiety, catastrophization, and so forth). Moreover, a history of trauma (including surgery) is frequently reported as a precipitating factor of the disease.[24] In this regard, CPSP may be part of these hypervigilant diseases unmasked in a vulnerable population by the preoperative stress and/or by surgery itself.

Circumstances linked to the anesthetic paradigm may help to turn physiologic into pathologic hyperalgesia. Large doses of synthetic opioids are administered during anesthesia, and it is now well recognized that opioids induce short-lasting analgesia and long-lasting hyperalgesia. This effect is demonstrated in various animal models and numerous clinical settings, including the anesthetic paradigm.[25] This effect shares common mechanisms (excitatory neurotransmission) with trauma-induced hyperalgesia. In normal or nonanesthetic circumstances, this opiate-induced hyperalgesia is of critical importance to preserve homeostasis in stress conditions. Opioid contributes to maintaining the balance between hypoalgesic and hyperalgesic processes and between the proinflammatory and antiinflammatory mediators.[25] During surgery, the dose of opioids administered for anesthetic purposes is totally disproportionate in regard to the amount of endogenous opiates physiologically required. Consequently, in addition to trauma-induced hyperalgesia, patients are exposed to significant opioid-induced hyperalgesia. At present, there is, however, no direct demonstration that this opioid-induced hyperalgesia favors the development of CPSP.

CPSP is probably the result of a deregulation of the mechanisms underlying secondary hyperalgesia. Why this deregulation occurs is still under debate. The factors leading to this deregulation are probably related to the patients (proinflammatory vulnerability or pathologic discrimination process) and circumstances (procedures associated with neuronal damages or determining important inflammatory reactions, drug-induced hyperalgesia).

Because prevention is the cornerstone of the treatment of CPSP, it is therefore important to underline the patients and circumstances associated with the development of this syndrome.

WHO DEVELOPS CPSP
Risk Factors

The main risk factors are summarized in **Box 2**.

Because only a fraction of the surgical patients develop CPSP, it is important to detect these patients before surgery. Several predictive factors for CPSP have been identified, which are related to both surgery and patients.

Factors linked to surgery are obvious when considering the previous section. These factors include invasive procedures, redo interventions, long-lasting surgery, and surgery in a previously injured area.[26] Using an animal model for chronic postthoracotomy pain, Buvanendran and colleagues[27] showed that a 60-minute rib retraction produced an incidence of 50% of long-term allodynia. In contrast, a 5- or 30-minute rib retraction

---

Box 2
Risk factors of developing CPSP

1. Type of surgery
2. Genetic predisposition
3. Female gender
4. Young age
5. Preoperative anxiety
6. Negative psychosocial factors
7. Obesity
8. Preexisting pain
9. Inflammatory state
10. Severe/poorly controlled postoperative pain

produced only an incidence of 10% of allodynia. In other words, all the surgical circumstances associated with important inflammatory reactions and damage to the nerve tissues are favoring factors.

Factors linked to the patients include the genetic background of the patient. It is well recognized that concerning pain perception and metabolism of analgesic drugs, the genetic polymorphism of the population is important. In this regard, there are some protective genotypes (homozygous carriers of a GTP cyclohydrolase I haplotype)[28] or phenotypes (children born of mothers with a familial history of hypertension, schizophrenia).[29,30] Nevertheless, according to the complexity of the mechanisms involved in pain perception, the recently isolated favorable haplotypes are not necessarily protective against all types of hyperalgesias (eg, somatic, visceral).[31] At present, the development of this area of study is still inadequate to allow systematic genotype screening to identify populations at risk of developing CPSP.

Gender: Female patients report greater level of pain after acute surgical procedures (moderate intensity of pain in 84% women vs 57% men). CPSP in female population occurs at a ratio greater than 2:1 when compared with men.[3]

Age: Young surgical patients are more prone to develop CPSP. Despite the fact that elderly patients have no significant modifications in pain thresholds and that peripheral neuropathies increase with aging, older age seems protective.[3]

Preoperative anxiety and/or catastrophization and negative psychosocial conditions: Preoperative anxiety has been identified to predispose to more intense postoperative pain during the first day after surgery.[32] High preoperative scores for anxiety, catastrophization personalities, and negative psychosocial situations are factors regularly reported in the history of patients suffering invalidating CPSP.[4,5,33]

Obesity: In the light of recent data, it is clear that the role of adipose tissue has changed from a lipid storage to an endocrine and immunoactive organ.[9] Modifications of the proinflammatory/antiinflammatory balance in obese patients favors the development of CPSP.[34,35]

The 3 following situations are also frequently found in the history of patients presenting with CPSP:

- Preexisting pain (not necessarily related to the surgical site)
- A history of an inflammatory process in the area of surgery[18]
- Conditions such as irritable bowel syndrome, migraine headache, fibromyalgia, and Raynaud disease.[36]

These situations are in accordance with the hypothesis of an algesic proinflammatory priming necessary for the development of CPSP.[22] In this regard, prospective studies would be interesting to confirm that neonatal surgery probably leads to increased pain sensitivity in later childhood and to residual pain.[37]

One of the most striking predictive factors of CPSP is the intensity of acute postoperative pain. Patients suffering intense postoperative pain are more prone than others to develop CPSP.[38–40]

In other words, the risk to intense acute postoperative is similar to that of CPSP.

STRATEGIES FOR PREVENTION

That the intensity of acute postoperative pain is a predictive factor for chronic pain is of critical importance for anesthetists. One of the first preventive measures is an adequate treatment of acute postoperative pain.

However, large surveys considering the efficacy of the treatment of acute postoperative pain revealed that the treatment remains inadequate. Dolin and colleagues,[41] in a cohort of 20,000 patients from published data, reported that 41% of patients experience moderate to severe pain after surgery. These data are confirmed in a national survey done by Apfelbaum and colleagues.[42] These investigators demonstrated that 31% of patients had severe or extreme pain and another 47% had moderate pain after surgery.

How to Improve the Treatment of Acute Postoperative Pain to Prevent CPSP

Before surgery, it is important to detect patients likely to suffer intense postoperative pain. Patients do not equally face pain; there exists a large interindividual variability in pain sensitivity and response to analgesic medications. Sensitive patients deserve specific treatment. This distinction is also of critical importance to evaluate the efficacy of these specific treatments.

A simple way to detect these patients at the preoperative visit is to fulfill the Kalkman score, a validated risk scale based on patient's history and the type of surgery (**Box 3**).[43,44]

Other investigators have developed more sophisticated tools to detect at-risk patients. These investigators elaborated testing based on experimental pain. In this regard, psychophysical measures exploring static pain parameters (pain thresholds, magnitude estimation of suprathreshold nociceptive stimuli, and tolerance) have been regularly reported to predict the intensity of acute postoperative pain in the early phase of an injury.[45] Nevertheless, these measures of response to an acute, phasic, experimental stimulus are less indicative of the complex pain modulation process that occurs after surgery. Some aspects of such modulation can be quantified by using the dynamic psychophysical measures of temporal summation and evocation of diffuse noxious inhibitory control, a measure recently reported to predict the risk of CPSP after thoracotomy.[46] In contrast with the Kalkman score, these tests are time consuming and resource consuming and therefore not easy to perform in daily clinical practice.

Box 3
Preoperative prediction of severe postoperative pain according to Kalkman and colleagues[43]

- Sex: female, 1 point; male, 0 point
- Age: younger than 30 years, 2 points; 31 to 65 years, 1 point; older than 65 years, 0 point
- Pain before surgery at the site: none, 0 point; moderate, 2 points; sévère, 3 points
- Regular use of opioids, 1 point
- Regular use of anxiolytic antidepressants, 1 point (otherwise 0)
- Open surgery, 1 point (otherwise 0)
- Type of surgery: thoracic, 3 points; abdominal, 2 points; orthopedic, 1 point; other, 0 point
- Long-lasting procedures (>120 minutes), 1 point (otherwise 0)
- Obesity (BMI>30), 1 point (otherwise 0)
- High level of anxiety at the preoperative visit, 1 point (otherwise 0)

The risk-intense postoperative pain is important when the score is 4 out of 15.

Data from Kalkman CJ, Visser K, Moen J, et al. Preoperative prediction of severe postoperative pain. Pain 2003;105:415–23; and Janssen K, Kalkman CJ, Grobbee DE, et al. The risk of severe postoperative pain: modification and validation of a clinical prediction rule. Anesth Analg 2008;107:1330–9.

Once these sensitive patients are detected at the preoperative visit, the anesthetists may help these patients to prepare themselves for surgery and postoperative pain. One way is to assist the patient to face the psychological stress associated with the surgery and its consequences. It is already mentioned that preoperative anxiety plays an important role in the intensity of postoperative pain, and anxious/catastrophizing personalities are factors recognized to favor CPSP.[32] Techniques to alleviate these negative mental statuses, such as autohypnotic conditioning, may certainly help.[47] However, these techniques deserve confirmation by prospective studies.

Another way is preoperative prehabilitation programs such as those used for fast-track procedures, including, among others, exercise rehabilitation.[48]

Moreover, light physical exercise may induce an inflammatory preconditioning that protects against exacerbated inflammatory stress consecutive to surgery.[49]

These 2 approaches implicate that the preoperative visit by the anesthetist occurs several weeks before surgery and that specialized facilities are available.

In the operating theater, prevention of CPSP is based on protective surgery and protective anesthesia/analgesia.

PROTECTIVE SURGERY

Acute postoperative pain and CPSP are linked to the surgical procedure. Therefore, it is judicious to speculate that surgery preserving nerve roots and producing minimal inflammatory reactions reduces the intensity of severe acute pain and the incidence of CPSP. This speculation was confirmed for groin hernia repair when techniques preserving nerves or materials inducing reduced inflammatory reaction were used.[50] No significant differences were, however, noted when open surgery was compared with laparoscopic approach.[51] Nevertheless, minimally invasive procedures should be recommended when applicable.

PROTECTIVE ANESTHESIA AND ANALGESIA

A critical question is whether anesthetic techniques can significantly influence the development of CPSP. Divergent opinions are found in the literature. Some investigators are convinced that surgery is the major determinant[50] and, consequently, that anesthetic techniques have little influence. Nevertheless, even if there exists no large prospective trial demonstrating that any specific anesthetic intervention reduces the risk of CPSP, anesthetic interventions can strongly influence the intensity of acute postoperative pain. Remember that acute postoperative pain intensity is an important determinant of the development of CPSP. In a cohort of patients recovering from general anesthesia, Aubrun and colleagues[52] reported that an important predictive factor of the severity of postoperative pain in the postanesthesia care unit is the dose of intraoperative opioids administered. Administration of intraoperative opioids promotes opiate-induced hyperalgesia with the consequence of increased postoperative pain.[53] To avoid this iatrogenic increase in the intensity of postoperative pain, anesthetists have to adopt opioid-sparing or opioid-protective anesthesia techniques. Opioids were introduced in the anesthetic paradigm in the mid-1960s mainly for their hemodynamic stabilizing effects and secondarily (incidentally) for their anesthetic-sparing properties.[54] At present, numerous alternatives are available for opioid sparing, that is, considering either nonanesthetic hemodynamic stabilizing drugs (ie, β-blockers) or anesthetic-sparing drugs, such as α_2-adrenergic agonists and combined locoregional/general anesthetic techniques. Moreover, ketamine, the dissociative anesthetic administered at antihyperalgesic dose, specifically protects against the hyperalgesic effects of opioids (see later).[55]

When considering specifically pain chronicization, the authors and other investigators have demonstrated, in a limited series of patients, that potent analgesia achieved with locoregional techniques combined with antihyperalgesic medications influences positively secondary surgery-related hyperalgesia and significantly reduces the incidence of CPSP after open colic surgery or thoracotomy.[12,18–56]

Before the anesthetic/analgesic strategies suspected to improve the incidence of CPSP can be detailed, 2 important remarks concerning the design of pain studies in the perioperative period are mandatory. In most cases, the choice of the studied population is based on a particular group of interventions or the type of surgery (gynecological, orthopedic procedures, or colectomy) and not on a particular risk. But for postoperative pain, some patients are more prone to suffer intense pain than others. Nevertheless, in many pain studies, the population recruited in the study was a mix of patients with different risk factors. This mixed recruitment introduces a serious flaw in the design of the study and thus the results.

In all the studies evaluating a drug or a technique to improve postoperative pain treatment, a precise evaluation of the specific pain risk of the patients (ie, using the Kalkman scale) should be presented to get an objective idea of the efficacy in the most-concerned population. The fact that this pain risk is not considered in the design of the studies may certainly account for the discrepancies found in the literature concerning the efficacy of various drugs and techniques. On the other hand, much attention is prompted on secondary hyperalgesia as an important determinant of CPSP. At present, how many studies on postoperative pain management consider parameters specific to secondary hyperalgesia?

Most studies in patients use the pain visual analog scale scores and/or a reduction in rescue (morphine patient-controlled analgesia) analgesic requirements as end points. These parameters do not measure secondary hyperalgesia or do so indirectly. The specific signs of secondary hyperalgesia, that is, the measurements of the area of hyperalgesia,[57] are quasi-never considered except in rare series. Moreover, prospective studies including an evaluation of a drug on the development of CPSP are particularly sparse when considering the mass of the data available on postoperative pain management. It is therefore not accurate to exclude any influence of analgesic techniques on CPSP because it is simply not known.

What is Protective Anesthesia/Analgesia

The aim of protective analgesia is to maximally reduce the importance of primary and secondary hyperalgesias, that is, to maximally reduce the excitatory input coming from the damaged periphery to the central nervous system and to put the central nervous system in a limited reactive state. For this purpose, it is advocated to use potent analgesic techniques combined with antihyperalgesics or drugs acting specifically on secondary hyperalgesia aimed at preventing the sensitization of the central nervous system, hence, to reduce the development of pathologic residual pain after surgery.[58,59]

What does potent analgesic techniques mean

In the context of prevention of intense acute postoperative pain and CPSP, it is clear that multimodal analgesia is mandatory. In this regard, the locoregional techniques are particularly interesting. These techniques provide a robust blockade of conduction for the influx of impulses arising from the injured area.[60] This blockade is, however, not sufficient to exclude any risk of CPSP. A meta-analysis including 458 patients (6 studies) failed to demonstrate significant difference in the incidence of chronic pain at 6 months with or without epidural technique.[61] This failure can easily be explained by the fact that locoregional techniques have little influence on the excitatory inputs mediated by the proinflammatory factors released at the site of injury.

In the absence of contraindications, nonsteroidal antiinflammatory drugs (NSAIDS) have to be considered as part of a multimodal analgesic approach.[62] Products of arachidonic metabolism promote pain and hyperalgesia associated with tissue trauma and inflammation. Inflammation causes a widespread induction of cyclooxygenase (COX) 2 in the spinal cord neurons and other regions of the central nervous system elevating prostaglandin E_2 (PGE_2) levels in the cerebrospinal fluid. PGE_2 is a key mediator of both peripheral and central pain sensitizations.[63] NSAIDS, by COX inhibition, help to alleviate acute pain and probably influence the development of CPSP. In a retrospective study considering postthoracotomy neuralgia, Richardson and colleagues[64] reported an incidence of chronic postthoracotomy pain of 23.4% in patients treated for early postoperative pain with opioids alone versus 14.8% in patients benefiting from paravertebral blocks. The incidence decreased to 9.9% when NSAIDS were added. Of interest are the perspectives offered by the new class of analgesic substances acting on the peripheral nociceptors *TRPV1* (transient receptor potential vanilloid type 1).[65] These receptors are ionic channels located preferentially on sensory nerves that are activated by chemical ligands, such as capsaicin or resiniferatoxin; protons; and heat. These receptors participate in the nociceptive perception consecutive to chemical, thermal, and mechanical stimuli and are also responsible for the neurogenic inflammation by releasing proinflammatory mediators (calcitonin gene-related peptide, cholecystokinin, substance P) from the nerve. Substances acting on these receptors are awaited not only to block the nociceptives inputs immediately at the site of its generation but also to interfere very early with the trauma-induced proinflammatory reactions.[66,67] Clinical studies with highly purified forms of capsaicin instilled in the surgical wound at the end of procedure (groin hernia repair, total knee prosthesis) confirmed the lack of toxicity but reported only a modest positive effect on early postoperative pain.[68,69]

Opioids remain the cornerstone of postoperative analgesia. These drugs are particularly efficient to alleviate primary hyperalgesia (spontaneous pain).[70,71] As already mentioned, opioids induce short-lasting analgesia and long-lasting hyperalgesia. This opiate-induced hyperalgesia is also under the dependence of the excitatory neurotransmission.[12,55] Therefore, to prevent this condition, it is logical to associate an opioid with an antagonist of the excitatory neurotransmission (NMDA receptor), such as ketamine.[72] Moreover, there is evidence to suggest that morphine is associated with a better recovery profile than other synthetic opioids, such as fentanyl. Morphine, in contrast to the synthetic one, binds to the µ3 receptor (alkaloid specific) that is involved in the regulation of the inflammatory reaction[73] and may account for the positive effects on early postoperative rehabilitation observed in patients undergoing coronary artery bypass graft under morphine compared with fentanyl analgesia.[74]

ANTIHYPERALGESICS, DRUGS ACTING ON SECONDARY HYPERALGESIA

Several drugs are particularly effective in preventing secondary hyperalgesia (**Box 4**). These drugs are reported experimentally and/or clinically to reduce evoked (mobilization) pain, area of hyperalgesia surrounding the wound, and, for some, the incidence of CPSP. Most drugs are not potent analgesics for primary hyperalgesia or spontaneous pain or are even devoid of any analgesic effect. The authors focus on the most representative of these drugs.

Ketamine is the prototype drug to be used as the antihyperalgesic in the perioperative period. This drug is active against opioid- and trauma-induced hyperalgesias.

Box 4
Drugs or substances showing antihyperalgesic effects

- Ketamine/memantine/magnesium
- Gabapentin-pregabalin
- COX-1/2 inhibitors
- α_2-adrenoceotor agonists (perimedullary)
- Free radical scavengers (mannitol, vitamin C, and so forth)
- N_2O, systemic local anesthetics
- Drugs active against glial activity (minoxidil, propentofylline)
- Diet enriched with omega-3 or others

Ketamine reduces the incidence of postoperative residual pain.[6,56,57,75] It is a competitive inhibitor at the NMDA site of the excitatory glutaminergic transmission. Excitatory neurotransmission is involved in the propagation and amplification of nociceptive inputs at central site.[76,77] Ketamine is also documented to be an antiproinflammatory substance and helps to restore inflammatory homeostasis in the case of trauma and sepsis. Ketamine specifically reduces the production of proinflammatory cytokines by interaction with their nuclear transcription precursor the nuclear factor κB by a specific action on the purinergic receptors (adenosine 2A) and/or a reinforcement of the anti-inflammatory cholinergic reflex.[78–80] This property is original and not directly related to its antagonism at the NMDA receptor. This occurrence may explain why better results are obtained with ketamine than with other NMDA antagonists, such as magnesium.[81] The dose of ketamine required for the antihyperalgesic effect are significantly smaller (0.1–0.5 mg/kg ± 1–2 μg/kg/min during 48–72 hours) compared with the doses used for anesthesia.[72] Moreover, the antiproinflammatory effect of ketamine after one dose is particularly prolonged.

Ketamine is considered as an important element of the protective analgesic techniques, although this characteristic is not obvious in the meta-analysis evaluating the role of ketamine in postoperative analgesia[82,83] possibly because these meta-analyses are based on studies considering only the efficacy of this drug on primary hyperalgesia.

Gabapentin and pregabalin are 2 promising drugs under evaluation as antihyperalgesics in the perioperative period. Gabapentin and pregabalin are alkylated γ-aminobutyric acid analogues that were first developed clinically as anticonvulsants. These drugs are active in the treatment of chronic neuropathic pain. They bind to the α2/δ subunits of voltage-gated calcium channels, thus preventing the release of nociceptive transmitters, including glutamate substance P and noradrenalin.[84] Despite some discordant results, several works report reduced incidence of chronic pain after surgery with the use of these drugs.[85–87]

These discrepancies are probably the result of a selection not taking into account population with comparable risk to develop CPSP.

The α_2-adrenoceptor agonists are interesting drugs to consider for multimodal analgesia and antihyperalgesia. Given by systemic route, these drugs potentiate the analgesic effects of the opioids (by a factor 4) without increasing their hyperalgesic properties.[88] Given by the spinal route, these drugs significantly reduce the area of secondary hyperalgesia when compared with bupivacaine or placebo and lower the incidence of CPSP after colonic surgery.[19] These effects are explained by the mechanism of action of the α_2-adrenoceptor agonists. These drugs mimic the effect of the central descending inhibitory controls on pain perception, silencing the interneurons involved in the windup phenomenon.[89]

Recently, promising results are reported from drugs acting as glial modulator, such as propentofylline, a methylxanthine derivative. Raghavendra and colleagues[90] have shown that chronic propentofylline treatment in neuropathic rats attenuated the development of hyperalgesia and restored the analgesic efficacy of morphine. Propentofylline inhibits glial activation and enhances spinal proinflammatory cytokines after peripheral nerve injury. Moreover, in animals, modulation of glial and neuroimmune activations may restore the analgesic efficacy of morphine in the treatment of neuropathic pain.[91]

SUMMARY

Postinjury hyperalgesia is a physiologic phenomenon. In the perioperative period, for unknown reasons (at-risk populations, exacerbated proinflammatory process, anesthetics- and/or analgesics-induced pathologic hyperalgesia), this phenomenon can be deregulated, leading to CPSP. Large prospective epidemiologic studies are mandatory to determine the exact incidence, favoring factors, and effect of the different anesthetic techniques of this phenomenon.

Prevention of CPSP is of critical concern for the anesthetist because, once established, it is as invalidating and difficult to treat as many other chronic pain conditions.

For this purpose, it is important to identify preoperatively patients who are prone to develop CPSP. Preoperative mental and physical preparations for the surgical stress should be initiated when possible. Protective surgical and anesthetic techniques, that is, techniques that avoid trauma to nerves, with reduced inflammatory stimuli, should be chosen. It is important to avoid the potential for opioid-induced hyperalgesia with the use of analgesic treatment combining potent analgesics and efficacy-proven antihyperalgesics.

For anesthetists it is important to follow-up the effect of such strategies on the occurrence of CPSP for both short and long terms. This follow-up helps to identify the onset of CPSP early and initiate the early treatment of patients with CPSP and to validate the efficacy of the preventive strategies.

REFERENCES

1. Macrae WA, Davies HT. In: Crombie IK, editor. Epidemiology of pain. Seattle (WA): IASP Press; 1999. p. 125–42.
2. Dajczman E, Gordon A, Kreisman H, et al. Long-term post-thoracotomy pain. Chest 1991;99:270–4.
3. Kelhet H, Jensen T, Woolf C. Persistent post surgical pain: risk factors and prevention. Lancet 2006;367:1618–25.
4. Gerbershagen HJ, Dagtekin O, Rothe T, et al. Risk factors for acute and chronic postoperative pain in patients with benign and malignant renal disease after nephrectomy. Eur J Pain 2009;13:853–60.
5. Gerbershagen H, Ozgur E, Dagtekin O, et al. Preoperative pain as a risk factor for chronic post-surgical pain—six month follow up after radical prostatectomy. Eur J Pain 2009;13:1054–61.
6. De Kock M, Lavand'homme P, Waterloos H. "Balanced analgesia" in the perioperative period: is there a place for ketamine? Pain 2001;92:373–80.
7. Crombie IK, Davies HT, Macrae WA. Cut and thrust: antecedent surgery and trauma among patients attending a chronic pain clinic. Pain 1998;76:167–71.

8. American Academy of Allergy, Asthma & Immunology. Asthma statistics. Available at: http://www.aaai.org/media/resources/media_kit/astma_statistics.stm. Accessed April 4, 2011.
9. Schaffler A, Scholmerich J. Innate immunity and adipose tissue biology. Trends Immunol 2010;31:226–35.
10. Eisenach JC. Preventing chronic pain after surgery: who, how, and when? Reg Anesth Pain Med 2006;31:1–3.
11. Milligan E, Watkins L. Pathological and protective role of glia in chronic pain. Nat Rev Neurosci 2009;10:22–36.
12. Angst MS, Clark JD. Opioid-induced hyperalgesia: a qualitative systemic review. Anesthesiology 2006;104:570–87.
13. Matta JA, Cornett PM, Miyares RL, et al. General anesthetics activate a nociceptive ion channel to enhance pain and inflammation. Proc Natl Acad Sci U S A 2008;105:8784–9.
14. Woolf CJ, Salter MW. Neuronal plasticity: increasing the gain in pain. Science 2000;288:1765–9.
15. Woolf CJ, Thompson SW. The induction and maintenance of central sensitization is dependent on N-methyl-D-aspartic acid receptor activation; implications for the treatment of postinjury hypersensitivity states. Pain 1991;44:293–9.
16. Coderre TZ, Katz J, Vaccario AL, et al. Contribution of central neuroplasticity to pathological pain: review of clinical and experimental evidence. Pain 1993;52:259–85.
17. Lavand'homme P, De Kock M, Waterloos H. Intraoperative epidural analgesia combined with ketamine provides effective preventive analgesia in patients undergoing major digestive surgery. Anesthesiology 2005;103:813–20.
18. Lavand'homme P, Roelants F, Waterloos H, et al. Postoperative analgesic effects of continuous wound infiltration with diclofenac after elective cesarean delivery. Anesthesiology 2007;106:1220–5.
19. De Kock M, Lavand'homme P, Waterloos H. The short-lasting analgesia and long-term antihyperalgesic effect of intrathecal clonidine in patients undergoing colonic surgery. Anesth Analg 2005;101:566–72.
20. Steegers M, Snik D, Verhagen A, et al. One half of the chronic pain after thoracic surgery shows a neuropathic component. J Pain 2008;10:955–61.
21. Jaaskelainen SK, Teerijoki-Osaka T, Virtanen A, et al. Sensory regeneration following intraoperatively verified trigeminal nerve injury. Neurology 2004;62:1951–7.
22. Omoigui S. The biochemical origin of pain—proposing a new law of pain: the origin of all pain is inflammation and the inflammatory response—a unifying law of pain. Med Hypotheses 2007;69:70–82.
23. Hollins M, Harper D, Gallagher S, et al. Perceived intensity and unpleasantness of cutaneous and auditory stimuli: an evaluation of the generalized hypervigilance hypothesis. Pain 2009;141:215–21.
24. White KP, Carette S, Harth M, et al. Trauma and fibromyalgia: is there an association and what does it means? Semin Arthritis Rheum 2000;29:200–16.
25. Stefano GB, Kream R. Endogenous opiates, opioids, and immune function: evolutionary brokerage of defensive behaviors. Semin Cancer Biol 2008;18:190–8.
26. Perkins FM, Kelhet H. Chronic pain as an outcome from surgery. A review of predictive factors. Anesthesiology 2000;93:1123–33.
27. Buvanendran A, Kroin JS, Kerns JM, et al. Characterization of a new animal model for evaluation of persistent post-thoracotomy pain. Anesth Analg 2004;99:1453–60.

28. Tegeder I, Costigan M, Griffin RS, et al. GTP cyclohydrolase and tetrahydrobiopterin regulate pain sensitivity and persistence. Nat Med 2006;12:1269–77.
29. France CR, Taddio A, Shah VS, et al. Maternal family history of hypertension attenuates neonatal pain. Pain 2009;142:189–93.
30. Murthy B, Narayan B, Nayagam S. Reduced perception of pain in schizophrenia; its relevance to the clinical diagnosis of compartment syndrome. Injury 2004;35: 1192–3.
31. Lazarev M, Lamb J, Barmada MM, et al. Does the pain-protective GTP cyclohydrolase haplotype significantly alter the pattern or severity of pain in humans with chronic pancreatitis? Mol Pain 2008;4:58–62.
32. Granot M, Ferber SG. The roles of pain catastrophizing and anxiety in the prediction of postoperative pain intensity: a prospective study. Clin J Pain 2005;21: 439–45.
33. Chatterjee S, Nan R, Fleshner N, et al. Permanent flank bulge is a consequence of flank incision for radical nephrectomy in one half of the patients. Urol Oncol 2004;22:36–9.
34. Miller FK, Merritt SA, Klauber-dermore N, et al. Acute and persistent postoperative pain after breast surgery. Pain Med 2009;10:708–15.
35. Okifuji A, Donaldson G, Barck L, et al. Relationship between fibromyalgia and obesity in pain, function, mood, and sleep. J Pain 2010;11:1329–37.
36. Joshi I, Ogunnaike BO. Consequences of inadequate pain relief and chronic persistent postoperative pain. Anesthesiol Clin North America 2005;23:21–36.
37. Peters J, Schouw R, Anand K, et al. Does neonatal surgery lead to increased pain sensitivity in later childhood. Pain 2005;114:444–54.
38. Katz J, Jackson M, Kavanagh B, et al. Acute pain after thoracic surgery predicts long term post-thoracotomy pain. Clin J Pain 1996;12:50–5.
39. Gotoda Y, Kambara N, Skai T, et al. The morbidity, time course and predictive factors for persistent post-thoracotomy pain. Eur J Pain 2001;5:89–96.
40. Gehling M, Scheidt CE, Niebergall H, et al. Persistent pain after elective trauma surgery. Acute Pain 1999;2:110–4.
41. Dolin SJ, Cashman JN, Bland JM. Effectiveness of acute postoperative pain management: I. Evidence from published data. Br J Anaesth 2002;89:409–23.
42. Apfelbaum JL, Chen C, metha SS, et al. Postoperative pain experience from a national survey suggests postoperative pain continues to be undermanaged. Anesth Analg 2003;97:534–40.
43. Kalkman CJ, Visser K, Moen J, et al. Preoperative prediction of severe postoperative pain. Pain 2003;105:415–23.
44. Janssen K, Kalkman CJ, Grobbee DE, et al. The risk of severe postoperative pain: modification and validation of a clinical prediction rule. Anesth Analg 2008;107: 1330–9.
45. Granot M, Lowenstein L, Yarnitsky D, et al. Postcaeseraen section pain prediction by experimental pain assessment. Anesthesiology 2003;98:1422–6.
46. Yarnitsky D, Crispel Y, Eisenberg E, et al. Prediction of chronic post-operative pain: pre-operative DNIC testing identifies patients at risk. Pain 2008;138:22–8.
47. Restif AS. Self-hypnosis, a resource for children undergoing painful treatment. Soins Pediatr Pueric 2010;254:37–9.
48. Carli F, Charlebois P, Stein B, et al. Randomized clinical trial of prehabilitation in colorectal surgery. Br J Surg 2010;97:1187–97.
49. Stefano G, Esch T, Bilfinger T, et al. Proinflammation and preconditioning protection are part of a common nitric oxide mediated process. Med Sci Monit 2010;16: RA125–30.

50. Aasvang E, Kelhet H. Chronic postoperative pain: the case of inguinal herniorrhaphy. Br J Anaesth 2005;95:69–76.
51. Oefelein M, Bayazit Y. Chronic pain syndrome after laparoscopic radical nephrectomy. J Urol 2003;170:1939–40.
52. Aubrun F, Valade N, Coriat P, et al. predictive factors of severe postoperative pain in the postanesthetic care unit. Anesth Analg 2008;106:1535–41.
53. Chia YT, Liu K, Wang JJ, et al. Intraoperative high dose of fentanyl induces postoperative fentanyl tolerance. Can J Anaesth 1999;48:872–7.
54. Lowenstein E, Hallowell P, Levine FH, et al. Cardiovascular response to large doses of intravenous morphine in man. N Engl J Med 1969;281:1389–93.
55. Celerier E, Rivat C, Jun Y, et al. Long-lasting hyperalgesia induced by fentanyl in rats: preventive effect of ketamine. Anesthesiology 2000;92:465–72.
56. Suzuki M, Haraguiti S, Sugimoto K, et al. Low-dose ketamine potentiates epidural analgesia after thoracotomy. Anesthesiology 2006;105:111–9.
57. Stubhaug A, Breivik H, Eide PK, et al. Mapping of punctuate hyperalgesia around a surgical incision demonstrates that ketamine is a powerful suppressor of central sensitization to pain following surgery. Acta Anaesthesiol Scand 1997;41:1124–32.
58. Dahl JB, Mathiesen O, Moiniche S. "Protective premedication": an option with gabapentin and related drugs? A review of gabapentin and pregabalin in the treatment of postoperative pain. Acta Anaesthesiol Scand 2004;48:1130–6.
59. Bromley L. Pre-emptive analgesia and protective premedication: what is the difference? Biomed Pharmacother 2006;60:336–40.
60. Senturk M, Ozcan PE, Talu GK, et al. The effects of 3 different analgesic techniques on long-term postthoracotomy pain. Anesth Analg 2002;94:11–5.
61. Bong CL, Samuel M, Ng JM, et al. Effects of preemptive epidural analgesia on post-thoracotomy pain. J Cardiothorac Vasc Anesth 2005;19:786–93.
62. Ashburn MA, Caplan RA, Caert DB, et al. Practice guidelines for acute pain management in the perioperative setting. An updated report by the American Society of Anesthesiologist Task Force on Acute Pain Management. Anesthesiology 2004;100:1573–81.
63. Samad TA, Sapirstein A, Woolf CJ. Prostanoids and pain: unraveling mechanisms and revealing therapeutic targets. Trends Mol Med 2000;8:390–6.
64. Richardson J, Sabanathan S, Mearns AJ, et al. Post-thoracotomy neuralgia. Pain Clin 1994;7:87–97.
65. Wong G, Gavva N. Therapeutic potential of vanilloid receptor TRPV1 agonists and antagonists as analgesics: recent advances and setbacks. Brain Res Rev 2009;60:267–77.
66. Di Marzo V, Blumberg P, Szallasi A. Endovanilloid signaling in pain. Curr Opin Neurobiol 2002;12:372–9.
67. Kissin I. Vanilloid-induced conduction analgesia: selective, dose-dependent, long-lasting, with low level of potential neurotoxicity. Anesth Analg 2008;107:271–81.
68. Aasvang EK, Hansen JB, Malmstrom J, et al. The effect of wound instillation of a novel purified capsaicin formulation on postherniotomy pain: a double-blind randomised, placebo-controlled study. Anesth Analg 2008;107:282–91.
69. Aasvang EK, Hansen JB, Kelhet H. Late sensory function after intraoperative capsaicin wound instillation. Acta Anaesthesiol Scand 2010;54:224–31.
70. Zahn PK, Brennan TJ. Primary and secondary hyperalgesia in a rat model for human postoperative pain. Anesthesiology 1999;90:863–72.
71. Kawamata M, Watanabe H, Nishikawa K, et al. Different mechanisms of development and maintenance of experimental incision-induced hyperalgesia in human skin. Anesthesiology 2002;97:550–9.

72. Joly V, Richebe P, Guignard B, et al. Remifentanil-induced postoperative hyperalgesia and its prevention with small-dose ketamine. Anesthesiology 2005;103:147–55.
73. Stefano GB, Cadet P, Kream R, et al. The presence of endogenous morphine signaling in animals. Neurochem Res 2008;33:1933–9.
74. Murphy GL, Szokol JW, Marymont JH, et al. Morphine-based cardiac anesthesia provides superior early recovery compared to fentanyl in elective cardiac surgery patients. Anesth Analg 2009;109:311–9.
75. Remerand F, Tendre Ch Le, Baud A, et al. The early and delayed analgesic effects of ketamine after total hip arthroplasty: a prospective, randomized, controlled, double-blind study. Anesth Analg 2009;109:1963–7.
76. Oye I. Ketamine analgesia, NMDA receptors and the gates of perception. Acta Anaesthesiol Scand 1998;42:747–9.
77. Rabben T, Skjelbred P, Oye I. Prolonged analgesic effect of ketamine, an N-methyl-D-aspartate receptor inhibitor, in patients with chronic pain. J Pharmacol Exp Ther 1999;289:1060–6.
78. Mazar J, Rogachev B, Shaked G, et al. Involvement of adenosine in the antiinflammatory action of ketamine. Anesthesiology 2005;102:1174–81.
79. Shibakawa YS, Sasaki Y, Goshima Y, et al. Effects of ketamine and propofol on inflammatory responses of primary glial cell cultures stimulated with lipopolysaccharide. Br J Anaesth 2005;95:803–10.
80. Czura C, Rosas-ballina M, Tracey K. Cholinergic regulation of inflammation. In: Adler R, editor. Psychoneuroimmunology. Rochester (NY): Elsevier; 2006. p. 85–95.
81. Lysakowski C, Dumont L, Czarnetsky C, et al. Magnesium as an adjuvant to postoperative analgesia: a systematic review of randomized trials. Anesth Analg 2007;104:1532–9.
82. McCartney C, Sinha A, Katz J. A qualitative systemic review of the role of NMDA antagonists in preventive analgesia. Anesth Analg 2004;98:1385–400.
83. Bell RF, Dahl JB, Moore RA, et al. Peri-operative ketamine for acute post-operative pain: a quantitative and qualitative systematic review (Cochrane review). Acta Anaesthesiol Scand 2005;49:1405–28.
84. Gilron I. Is gabapentin a "broad spectrum" analgesic. Anesthesiology 2002;97:537–9.
85. Fassoulaki A, Triga A, Melemeni A, et al. Multimodal analgesia with gabapentin and local anesthetics prevents acute and chronic pain after breast surgery for cancer. Anesth Analg 2005;101:1427–32.
86. Buvanedran A, Kroin JS, Della Valle CJ, et al. Perioperative oral pregabalin reduces chronic pain after total knee arthroplasty: a prospective randomised, controlled trial. Anesth Analg 2010;110:199–207.
87. Arm Y, Yousef A. Evaluation of efficacy of the perioperative administration of venlafaxine or gabapentin on acute and chronic postmastectomy pain. Clin J Pain 2010;26:31–5.
88. Meert T, De Kock M. Potentiation of the analgesic properties of fentanyl-like opioids with α2-adrenoceptor agonists in rats. Anesthesiology 1994;81:678–88.
89. Eisenach J, De Kock M, Klimscha W. α2-adrenergic agonists for regional anesthesia: a clinical review of clonidine (1984–1995). Anesthesiology 1996;85:655–74.
90. Raghavendra V, Tanga F, Rutkowski M, et al. Anti-hyperalgesic and morphine-sparing actions of propentofylline following peripheral nerve injury in rats: mechanistic implications of spinal glia and pro-inflammatory cytokines. Pain 2003;104:655–64.
91. Song P, Zhao Z. The involvement of glial cells in the development of morphine tolerance. Neurosci Res 2001;39:281–6.

Local Infiltration Analgesia

Sugantha Ganapathy, MBBS, DA, FRCA, FFARCS (I), FRCPC[a,b,*],
Jonathan Brookes, FRCA[c], Robert Bourne, MD, FRCSC[d]

KEYWORDS

- Wound infiltration analgesia • Periarticular infiltration
- Local anesthetics • Fast track surgery
- Elastomeric infusion device

Pain after major abdominal, orthopedic, and thoracic surgeries can be significant resulting in unacceptable morbidity. Poorly controlled pain results in patient dissatisfaction and may also be associated with major morbidities, which includes perioperative myocardial ischemia, pulmonary complications, altered immune function, and postoperative cognitive dysfunction, to mention a few.[1,2] A variety of techniques are currently used to manage this pain, and opioids are amongst the most frequently used, either parenterally or neuraxially. Recent literature supports the use of regional anesthesia in the form of various peripheral nerve blocks as a better alternative (see the article by Brian Ilfeld elsewhere in this issue for further exploration of this topic). Whereas regional anesthesia for the upper limb can be provided with safety both in the hospital as well in the ambulatory setting,[3,4] lower limb regional blocks pose a particular problem of unpredictable motor blockade and the potential for falls.[5] On a similar note, although thoracic epidural analgesia provides excellent pain relief with improved outcomes particularly with regard to pulmonary complications[6] and

Conflict of Interest: S.G. has received funding from the Government of Ontario for her work on early discharge after arthroplasty. She has received support from I-Flow Corporation for her initial work on periarticular infiltration in kind contribution of infusion devices and financial support for measuring plasma local anesthetic levels.

[a] Department of Anesthesiology and Perioperative Medicine, University of Western Ontario, B3213, London Health Sciences Centre, University Hospital, 339 Windermere Road, London, Ontario N6A 5A5, Canada
[b] Department of Anesthesiology, Duke University Medical Centre, 2400 Pratt Street, # 311, Durham, NC 27705-3976, USA
[c] Schulich School of Medicine & Dentistry, University of Western Ontario, London, Ontario N6A 5C1, Canada
[d] Division of Orthopedics, Department of Surgery, Schulich School of Medicine & Dentistry, University of Western Ontario, London, Ontario N6A 5C1, Canada
* Corresponding author. Department of Anesthesiology and Perioperative Medicine, University of Western Ontario, B3213, London Health Sciences Centre, University Hospital, 339 Windermere Road, London, Ontario N6A 5A5, Canada.
E-mail address: Sugantha.Ganapathy@lhsc.on.ca

postoperative arrhythmia, it is associated with major undesirable side effects such as neuraxial hematoma or abscess. Thus, anticoagulation, sepsis, and spinal malformations can preclude the use of this elegant modality of analgesia in some patients. Most regional techniques require special expertise, a dedicated area to initiate them, and a trained coordinated team to provide postoperative management of the indwelling catheters. There is a need for alternate analgesic techniques to provide postoperative analgesia. The introduction of wound infiltration with local anesthetics not only provides this much-needed alternative analgesia but, in fact, in some cases, provides superior analgesia. At present, simple cost-effective analgesic techniques that provide improved outcomes for patients are needed. The techniques should be easy to administer and follow up. Wound infusions can be initiated by the surgeon at the end of surgery, with catheters inserted under direct vision. Are they as simple and effective as they seem? This article discusses the role and evidence for wound infiltration analgesia in general surgery, orthopedic surgery, neurosurgery, and thoracic surgery.

ABDOMINAL SURGERY

Abdominal surgery requires analgesia of not only the abdominal wall but also the viscera. Upper abdominal surgery is associated with significant pain during ambulation and breathing such that splinting of the diaphragm occurs unless adequate analgesia is provided. Although wound infiltration for abdominal analgesia was used as early as 1986,[7] it was not used to its full potential until the early nineties. In an earlier study, Hamid and colleagues[8] incorporated a continuous celiac plexus block with intermittent wound infiltration with local anesthetic, compared it with placebo, and noted that it reduced opioid requirement at 4 hours but did not provide acceptable level of analgesia. In a more recent elegant investigation, Beaussier and colleagues[9] noted that a preperitoneal infusion of ropivacaine at 10 mL/h reduced the diaphragm dysfunction compared with the placebo infusions given to a control group. Anecdotally, insertion of wound catheters on either side of the wound under the rectus sheath and infusion of local anesthetic at 2 mL per catheter per hour using an elastomeric pump provided good wound analgesia and reduced narcotic requirement but did not eliminate the need for narcotics. Although the method worked with primary laparotomies in the authors' experience, when patients came for reoperation, the tissue planes were rather difficult to identify and separate to appropriately position the catheters. There seems to be a difference in their efficacy between upper and lower abdominal surgeries. For postcesarean section analgesia, wound infiltration has been used more frequently with better outcomes. Bamigboye and Justus[10] used peritoneal and wound spraying of 30 mL of ropivacaine 0.75% after cesarean section and noted that the incidence of severe pain and narcotic and adjuvant analgesic requirement is reduced with this intervention. This intervention has been reviewed by the same investigators recently.[11] Mounir and colleagues[12] using bupivacaine wound infiltration after inguinal hernia repair found a reduction in acute pain during rest and coughing as well as a reduction in chronic postsurgical pain. Beaussier and colleagues[13] have also documented the efficacy of preperitoneal local anesthetic infusion for colorectal surgery. Additives such as magnesium[14] and tramadol have been documented to improve analgesia produced by local infiltration. Tauzin-Fin and colleagues,[14] in a randomized double-blind study, demonstrated a reduction of total cumulative tramadol consumption to 221 ± 64.1 mg in the group that received intravenous magnesium sulfate combined with ropivacaine infiltration and to 134 ± 74.9 mg in the group in which magnesium was added to ropivacaine for wound infiltration after radical retropubic prostatectomy. On the contrary, Berthon and colleagues[15] did not find that local anesthetic wound infiltration was beneficial in laparoscopic prostatectomy and advised that it should not be used routinely. One may suspect that perhaps the pain associated with minimally invasive surgery is significantly less to start with. Similarly, in a randomized, prospective, double-blind, placebo-controlled study in 68 patients, Updike and colleagues[16] infiltrated the incision site before abdominal hysterectomy with 30 mL of placebo or 0.5% ropivacaine. There was no difference between the groups with regard to pain scores or narcotic consumption at any time point. On the contrary, more recent studies using continuous wound infusions have shown that it provides better analgesia, reduces opioid consumption, and results in reduced duration of ileus and length of hospital stay with overall cost savings of €273 per patient.[17,18] The catheters were positioned in the transversus abdominis plane and subcutaneously, which implies that the catheter location is important for efficacy. In children, wound infiltration with local anesthetic performed either before incision or at the end of surgery resulted in less pain[19,20] and less stress response in the form of lower cortisol and prolactin levels in the group that received local anesthetic. The sample size in these studies is small, therefore further studies are needed to confirm these findings.[19]

TONSILLECTOMY

Infiltration of the tonsillar fossa or packing the fossa with local anesthetic–soaked gauze has been in use for several years to provide analgesia after tonsillectomy. Stelter and colleagues,[21] in a prospective randomized study in 180 subjects aged 3 to 45 years evaluated techniques of wound infiltration with patients acting as their own active comparator on the contralateral side. They compared 3 different techniques of depositing local anesthetic into the wound, preincisional infiltration, postincisional infiltration, and tonsillar fossa packing with bupivacaine-soaked gauze. Posttonsillectomy infiltration provided the best analgesia. This article is well referenced for the reader to get further information on this topic.

BREAST AND PLASTIC RECONSTRUCTIVE SURGERY

Local anesthetic infusion into the wound after the use of transverse rectus abdominal muscle flaps has been documented to produce better analgesia compared with placebo. Dagtekin and colleagues[22] infiltrated 20 mL of ropivacaine 0.2% followed by an infusion of 0.2% ropivacaine at 10 mL/h into the wound. The pain scores were better with ropivacaine infusion. It was also associated with earlier return of bowel function. Ropivacaine levels were also reported to be within therapeutic range. Ropivacaine in spite of its vasoconstrictive properties did not affect flap perfusion. The quality of recovery scores was significantly better in the ropivacaine group. Legeby and colleagues,[23] in a randomized placebo-controlled trial studied pain scores and narcotic consumption after breast reconstruction with repeated injections of local anesthetic into the wound via an indwelling catheter. Although the pain scores were better in the local anesthetic group in the first 24 hours, the opioid consumption was not different between the groups. On a larger scale, Pacik and colleagues[24] reported on a cohort of 644 patients over the course of 10 years who received either patient-administered boluses of local anesthetic into the wound or continuous infusion of local anesthetic using an elastomeric device after augmentation mammoplasty. Both techniques provided good analgesia for the first postoperative day, and no one developed local anesthetic toxicity. There was 1 wound infection that resulted in the loss of prosthesis. The investigators allowed patients to self administer 20 mL of 0.25% bupivacaine via an indwelling catheter into the wound once or twice more.

The investigators noted that the system of patient self-administration of local anesthetic into the wound was cheaper than the continuous infusion. Although no adverse events were documented, one must take into consideration the risk of intravascular injection of a total of 40 mL of bupivacaine if bilateral procedures are done, which could be lethal occurring late in the evening or early in the morning outside the hospital. Other investigators have not noted such a benefit with wound infiltration after breast surgery. Not all studies have found a similar benefit to wound infiltration after breast surgery,[25–27] certainly not when compared with paravertebral blocks. Similarly, for abdominoplasty, the results of wound infiltration and infusion have not been favorable.[28]

NEUROSURGERY

At the authors' institution, neurosurgeons have been infiltrating the scalp before surgery and head pinning for more than 20 years. Is there any evidence for its efficacy? In a recent study Saringcarinkul and Boonsri[29] noted that scalp infiltration provided only 1 hour of analgesia. Contrary to that, wound infiltration after back surgery seems to be effective, possibly related to vascularity and removal of local anesthetic from the site.[30] There are no data on continuous wound infusion in this area.

ORTHOPEDIC SURGERY

Continuous peripheral nerve blocks have been used to provide analgesia after both upper limb and lower limb orthopedic procedures. However, this procedure requires expertise and a dedicated team to initiate, maintain, and manage the blocks. There is also associated motor weakness with continuous regional analgesia, which can be managed with a sling with the upper limb, although many patients dislike the sensation of a weak floppy limb. With the lower limb, there is more than 1 group of nerves involved in carrying the sensation from the limb, necessitating dual regional blocks to provide adequate pain relief. The motor weakness poses additional risk in the form of falls and injuries.[5] Thus, many researchers in Europe and the continental United States were looking for equivalent analgesic techniques to provide postoperative pain relief after orthopedic surgery. Several investigators[31–38] have used intra-articular and periarticular infusions of bupivacaine for shoulder surgery, documented its efficacy against placebo as well as interscalene blocks, and found them to be effective. However, cases of chondrolysis after intra-articular infusion of bupivacaine were brought to the attention of the medical community.[39–41] It was noted that bupivacaine was chondrotoxic in animal experiments when infused into the shoulder joint.[42] It was also noted that the incidence of chondrolysis was higher with infusions higher than 2 mL/h.[43,44] This topic has been well reviewed in several articles published recently.[45–47] Many infusion device companies have issued specific warning with regard to intra-articular infusions.[48] There are several litigations across the United States for chondrolysis resulting from bupivacaine wound infusion into the shoulder joint. This chondrolysis may also be because the joint space is small and the local anesthetic concentration can build up resulting in chondronecrosis. Thus, at present, it is not advisable to use intra-articular infusions of local anesthetic into the shoulder joint. There has been no correlation noted with single injections at the end of surgery, and thus it is still common practice to use single postoperative injections into the soft tissues and subacromial area.

The situation with total joint arthroplasty of hip and knee is different because the cartilage would have been removed before implantation of prosthesis and thus there is no worry about chondronecrosis except in unicompartmental knee replacements. Kerr and Kohan[49] have done the initial work on wound infiltration in Sydney, Australia, since the early part of this decade, and they have published their ongoing work only recently. Although they did not publish their results until last year, many who visited their facility learned their technique and instituted it at their institution, including the authors' institution, and published on the efficacy of the intra-articular and periarticular infiltration analgesia. Their technique involved infiltrating the periarticular tissues in layers with a mixture of ropivacaine (total 300 mg in 150–200 mL), ketorolac, and epinephrine, 5 µg/mL. They positioned an epidural catheter anterior to the posterior capsule of the knee joint inserted to travel medial to the prosthesis through which they reinjected additional local anesthetic mixture when the patient complained of pain. All patients received multimodal analgesia using ibuprofen, acetaminophen, and low-dose narcotics. They had a standardized early-mobilization paradigm, avoided urinary catheterization, aggressively managed fluid status, and used only low-dose spinal anesthesia for surgery. They have reported on 325 patients managed using this paradigm and have managed to get the pain scores to less than 3 in more than 80% of patients during rest and activity during the first couple of days. They use only acetylsalicylic acid for deep vein thrombosis prophylaxis and enoxaparin only for specific indications. Elastocrepe bandages and icepacks were used to prolong the duration of locally injected drug. All patient interactions and reinjections occurred only with the surgeon and the specific anesthesiologist involved in their care, a luxury, which is difficult to deliver elsewhere. The only adverse event noted was dizziness on mobilization. Mauerhan and colleagues[50] could not show any benefit when the drugs were injected intra-articularly, but and Kerr and Kohan[49] have clearly shown the importance of soft tissue infiltration and an accelerated pathway of recovery. Although wound infiltration has been discussed by many in the past,[50–54] Kerr and Kohan[49] have genuinely stimulated the academic community to look at peripheral analgesia as a viable option, and this is highlighted by the editorial by Kehlet.[55]

Total Hip Arthroplasty

There are a few studies on the efficacy and safety of wound infiltration for analgesia after hip arthroplasty.[56,57] Anderson and colleagues[56] randomized 40 patients to receive wound infiltration with ropivacaine or placebo at the end of surgery followed by reinjection through an indwelling catheter with ropivacaine or placebo at 24 hours and studied analgesic efficacy and functional outcome. They observed that the patients who received the analgesic solution had less pain during rest and activity, less stiffness, and better Western Ontario and McMaster Universities Osteoarthritis Index (WOMAC) pain scale, function, and stiffness scores for 1 week postoperatively. Significant numbers of them were discharged home earlier, and many were very satisfied with the analgesic regime. More recently, Busch and colleagues[57] performed a randomized prospective study in which they included 64 patients to receive periarticular infiltration with a mixture of local anesthetic, ketorolac, and morphine or no infiltration and studied their postoperative pain scores and narcotic consumption. It was found that the intervention resulted in improved pain scores in the postanesthesia care unit associated with reduced narcotic consumption in the first 24 hours after surgery. The benefits of analgesia did not last beyond the first 24 hours, but their study is underpowered to draw conclusions on the long-term benefits of wound infiltration. The infiltration did not increase wound complications in this study.

Whether periarticular infusion improves analgesia for a longer period is as yet unknown. The authors studied the benefits of infusion initially in a small pilot study (SG and DGC, unpublished data, 2005). A set of 30 patients undergoing total hip arthroplasty (THA) were randomized to receive either periarticular wound infiltration with a mixture of ropivacaine, ketorolac, and morphine followed by an infusion of local anesthetic using multiorifice catheters or only multimodal analgesia followed by intravenous patient-controlled analgesia with morphine. The pain scores and narcotic consumption were significantly lower in the infiltration group but the benefit did not extend beyond the initial 24 hours after THA. This result is different from what the authors noted with total knee joint arthroplasty. Thus the benefits of infiltration are not prolonged by wound infusion of local anesthetic. This result could also be because of the image-guided THA that was done in the authors' patients, which required additional pins in the iliac crest and lower femur, areas that could be covered by additional infiltration but cannot be covered by infusion.

Total Knee Joint Replacement

The success with wound infusions and infiltrations is more obvious with total knee arthroplasty basically because the pain from this surgery seems significantly more compared with that from THA. Several studies from different countries[58–68] have documented the efficacy of wound infiltration with a variety of solutions, and an occasional one has documented the lack of efficacy of this technique[69] compared with peripheral nerve blocks as well. Whereas some earlier studies evaluated intra-articular infusion of local anesthetic and morphine to be ineffective for total knee joint arthroplasty,[50] recent studies[65,70] have documented the periarticular infusions and subcapsular infusions to provide superb analgesia. Some studies have documented the efficacy of single injection of periarticular infiltration,[59,63,66] whereas most others have documented the benefits of reinjection through an epidural catheter positioned anterior to the posterior capsule of knee joint 24 hours later.[58,60–62,64,65,67,68,70] Although many have reinjected through an indwelling intra-articular catheter, one must consider the risks of introducing infection with such reinjections via a newly implanted prosthesis. Considering the infection rate after arthroplasties is in the region of 0.5% to 1%, a large sample size is required to evaluate this complication. In one study, cultures were performed on the catheters after removal and 2 positive culture results were documented without evidence of joint infection, although low-grade infections might take months to become obvious. To avoid reinjecting through the catheter, the authors use a closed system of infusion using an elastomeric pump connected to the multiorifice catheters inserted by the surgeon at the end of surgery (SG and DGC, unpublished data, 2005). This infusion was continued for 48 hours. The authors' initial pilot study on 30 patients randomized to periarticular infiltration followed by infusion versus patient-controlled intravenous morphine analgesia revealed significant reduction in narcotic use and improved pain scores, with no motor blockade in either group. These patients had 1 catheter inserted percutaneously into the posterior knee fat pad, the second catheter subcapsularly in the suprapatellar pouch, and the third one subcutaneously and used 2 elastomeric pumps to deliver 2 mL per catheter per hour of 0.3% ropivacaine. This paradigm provided the best analgesia during the initial trials, allowing early ambulation on the day of surgery. The authors have since then performed another study in which they processed 100 patients (50 knees and 50 hips) and allowed them to get discharged 24 to 36 hours after surgery (unpublished data). They managed sending home 85% of the patients within 36 hours with good quality pain relief and no wound-related complications. Such early discharge does not entirely depend on wound infiltration and infusion alone but a whole paradigm of early rehabilitation, which this technique lends us to use.

Where do we put these catheters? The original description by Kerr and Kohan[49] talks about positioning the epidural catheter in the posterior knee inserted lateral to the anterior cruciate ligament (ACL), and later descriptions talk about positioning the catheter medial to the medial condyle of the femur. The authors have modified the technique to avoid the catheter getting caught between the condyles during ambulation. They insert a catheter posterior to the knee percutaneously connected to a single pump, and the intra-articular catheter is positioned in the suprapatellar pouch of the synovium (**Fig. 1**). The subcutaneous catheter and the intra-articular catheters are connected via a Y piece to a single pump (**Fig. 2**). This system allowed predictable analgesia to both the anterior and posterior compartments of the knee. The posterior catheter produced sciatic weakness below the knee in 1 patient, which resolved on holding the infusion for 4 hours, which allowed the surgeon to evaluate the sciatic function.

Toftdahl and colleagues[60] compared the wound infiltration followed by reinjection through the catheter at 24 hours with continuous femoral nerve block. They used a rather high concentration of ropivacaine in their femoral catheter and noted that the motor blockade from the block was significantly preventing ambulation. In the authors' experience, even with significantly lower concentrations of ropivacaine in the femoral catheters, there is variable quad weakness, increasing the risk of fall during ambulation. Compared with this, the authors found no motor weakness with periarticular infiltration/infusion, thus allowing the patient to ambulate as early as 4 hours after surgery.

Drugs Used

Although ropivacaine was the commonest reported because of its documented safety, many have used bupivacaine or levobupivacaine in its place with equal efficacy. The concentration of ropivacaine used varies from a large volume of 0.2% to a low volume of higher-concentration solutions with equal efficacy. The total dose used for infiltration is on an average 300 to 400 mg of ropivacaine. At their institution, the authors infiltrate with 300 mg of ropivacaine mixed with 30 mg of ketorolac, 2.5 µg/mL of epinephrine, and 10 mg of morphine. They have started adding morphine based on the basic science data on increased opiate receptor expression in wounds. Recent reports of analgesia through peripheral opiate receptor in the dental literature confirm the efficacy of this route of opiate administration for analgesia.[71,72] There are no prospective randomized trials to evaluate the role of morphine in the injectate. The authors have infused the wound continuously via multiorifice catheters with 0.35% ropivacaine with 2 mL/catheter/hour for a total of 6 mL/h for 48 hours. Often, patients had good analgesia for an additional day after termination of infusion.

More recently, steroids have been added to the infiltration mixture,[73,74] resulting in prolonged improvement in analgesia for as long as a week. This prolonged improvement may be attributable to the antiinflammatory effect of steroids locally. Whether

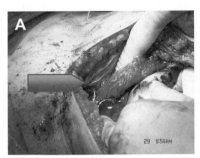
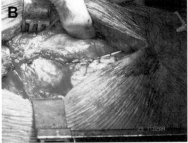

Fig. 1. (*A, B*) Intra-articular catheter positioned in the suprapatellar pouch in the knee (*arrow*) and subcutaneous catheter.

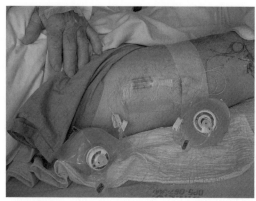

Fig. 2. Periarticular catheters connected to elastomeric pumps for total knee joint arthroplasty.

such use alters wound healing or predisposes to infective complications is still unknown because the number of patients is small. For one to find a difference in the infection rates, several hundred patients will have to be randomized. This requires further studies with regard to both efficacy and safety.

Infusion

While the cheapest way to infuse drugs into the wound is by using simple disposable epidural catheters inserted into the wound, when the authors attempted using such a system, the catheters often got clogged with local blood that could not be reinjected through the catheter. Other studies do not mention this problem. In addition, infusion through these catheters did not really cover the entire length of the incision. Thus the authors have resorted to the use of kits with multiorifice catheters. These catheters are currently marketed by several companies along with disposable elastomeric or spring-loaded infusion devices. Although these equipments are relatively expensive, they take away the worry of cross-contamination between patients as well as the worry of reinjection through an indwelling catheter apart from allowing the patients to be discharged home early with infusions at home. The report by Toftdahl and colleagues[60] document 3 patients who developed wound complications. They found that 2 patients had wound bullae and 1 required a gastrocnemius flap. Also, 1 patient had early infection, necessitating incision and drainage of the wound and poly exchange. One has to wonder if this may be related to the high concentration of epinephrine used in the infiltrate. The authors have studied the plasma ropivacaine levels in a small subset of patients (SG and colleagues, unpublished data, 2006) and noted that the plasma levels of ropivacaine were similar between the group that received epinephrine, 2.5 μg/mL, and the one that received epinephrine 5 μg/mL. Thus the authors currently use only 2.5 μg/mL of epinephrine in the infiltrate because ropivacaine is already vasoconstrictive. In the same study, Toftdahl and colleagues[60] reported adverse events during reinjection via the catheter in 2 patients, 1 developing chest pain and the second become transiently unconscious. The authors have seen a few complications in their series as well. They reported that 1 catheter got entangled in the cement and broke as it was withdrawn and was thus left in the wound. To date, there is no evidence of granuloma or infection 2 years later. One patient discharged home 24 hours after surgery after THA developed acute myocardial infarction at home on the third postoperative day. Three patients had postoperative neurologic deficits in the sciatic distribution, one of which was after a resurfacing THA and was prolonged but recovered completely. The second one was after a total knee arthroplasty in the form of tingling paresthesia transiently in the sciatic distribution but recovered within a week.

The authors think that these deficits are most likely needle injuries during infiltration, although retraction injury to the sciatic nerve with the resurfacing THA, which can be associated with a 1% incidence of postoperative sciatic dysfunction, cannot be ruled out. Kerr and Kohan[49] specifically recommends using a smaller-gauge spinal needle and inject as one moves the needle back and forth to prevent injecting into the vessels or, possibly, the nerves. The third patient in the authors' series had intermittent sciatic area weakness below the knee and developed heel blisters because of rubbing of the heel during physiotherapy.

Although the authors used multiorifice catheters, a recent study by Anderson and colleagues[75] notes no difference in the spread between epidural catheter and the multiorifice catheter positioned in the subfascial location after a THA. As suggested by these investigators, this topic needs to be evaluated in other areas as well and on a larger scale.

Advantages and Disadvantages

The principal advantage of wound infiltration technique is the ease of administration and follow-up, requiring no special expertise. The second major advantage is the lack of motor blockade. Its success depends on the meticulously executed infiltration by the surgeon. Although the team may supplement if needed in the recovery area similar to the Australian group, reinjection should not be taken lightly if there is a variety of caregivers taking part in the care of the patient. There is preliminary suggestion of a prolonged analgesia with this analgesic technique, which requires a larger prospective trial to confirm. There definitely is economic savings that can accrue from early discharge. At the authors' institution, with the lack of tertiary care beds, this is particularly useful. Even bilateral knee replacements have been done using this technique for analgesia.

The potential disadvantages include the potential for local anesthetic toxicity and wound complications. Many patients with wound infiltration and infusion after THA had episodes of dizziness, fainting, and low hemoglobin levels because of blood loss into the tissues. Thus, it is important to keep the patients well hydrated before ambulation is attempted. This technique is not for patients who are already taking large doses of narcotics with preexisting potential opioid-induced hyperalgesia. In environments in which the anesthesiologist billing for regional blocks forms a major contribution to their income, wound infusions may significantly modify the anesthesia income. Exposure to latex had been reported with certain elastomeric devices apart from unpredictable deliveries with certain devices.

SUMMARY

Wound infiltration and infusion of local anesthetics either alone or mixed with adjuvants provide excellent analgesia with potential for early discharge. The economic advantages with this technique should be explored further. This technique is particularly useful in situations in which other regional anesthetic techniques are either contraindicated or are not possible because of comorbities such as infection and coagulopathy.

REFERENCES

1. Joshi GP, Ogunnaike BO. Consequences of inadequate postoperative pain relief and chronic persistent postoperative pain. Anesthesiol Clin North America 2005; 23:21–36.

2. Liu SS, Wu CL. The effect of analgesic technique on postoperative patient reported outcomes including analgesia: a systematic review. Anesth Analg 2007; 105:789–808.

3. Ilfeld BM, Enneking FK. Continuous peripheral nerve blocks at home: a review. Anesth Analg 2005;100:1822–33.

4. Hanna MN, Murphy JD, Kumar K, et al. Regional techniques and outcome: what is the evidence? Curr Opin Anaesthesiol 2009;22:672–7.

5. Ilfeld BM, Duke KB, Donohue MC. The association between lower extremity continuous peripheral nerve blocks and patient falls after knee and hip arthroplasty. Anesth Analg 2010;111:1552–4.

6. Mankikian B, Cantineau JP, Bertrand M, et al. Improvement of diaphragmatic function by a thoracic extradural bloc after upper abdominal surgery. Anesthesiology 1988;68:379–86.

7. Levack I, Holmes J, Robertson G. Abdominal wound perfusion for the relief of postoperative pain. Br J Anaesth 1986;58:615–9.

8. Hamid SK, Scott NB, Sutcliffe NP, et al. Continuous coeliac plexus blockade plus intermittent wound infiltration with bupivacaine following upper abdominal surgery: a double-blind randomized study. Acta Anaesthesiol Scand 1992; 36(6):534–9.

9. Beaussier M, El'Ayoubi H, Rollin M, et al. Parietal analgesia decreases postoperative diaphragm dysfunction induced by abdominal surgery. A physiologic study. Reg Anesth Pain Med 2009;34:393–7.

10. Bamigboye AA, Justus HG. Ropivacaine abdominal wound infiltration and peritoneal spraying at cesarean delivery for preemptive analgesia. Int J Gynaecol Obstet 2008;102:160–4.

11. Bamigboye AA, Justus HG. Caesarean section wound infiltration with local anaesthesia for postoperative pain relief-any benefit? Suid-Afrikaanse Tydskrif Vir Geneeskunde. S Afr Med J 2010;100(5):313–9.

12. Mounir K, Bensghir M, Elmoqaddem A, et al. Efficiency of bupivacaine wound subfasciale infiltration in reduction of postoperative pain after inguinal hernia surgery. Ann Fr Anesth Reanim 2010;29(4):274–8 [in French].

13. Beaussier M, El'Ayoubi H, Schiffer E, et al. Continuous preperitoneal infusion of ropivacaine provides effective analgesia and accelerates recovery after colorectal surgery: a randomized, double-blind, placebo-controlled study. Anesthesiology 2007;107:461.

14. Tauzin-Fin P, Sesay M, Svartz L, et al. Wound infiltration with magnesium sulphate and ropivacaine mixture reduces postoperative tramadol requirements after radical prostatectomy. Acta Anaesthesiol Scand 2009;53:464–9.

15. Berthon N, Plainard X, Cathelineau X, et al. Effect of wound infiltration of ropivacaine in postoperative pain after extraperitoneal laparoscopic radical prostatectomy. Prog Urol 2010;20(6):435–9 [in French].

16. Updike GM, Manolistas TP, Cohn DE, et al. Pre-emptive analgesia in gynecologic surgical procedures: preoperative wound infiltration with ropivacaine in patients who undergo laparotomy through a midline vertical incision. Am J Obstet Gynecol 2003;188:901–5.

17. Gomez Rios MA, Vazquez Barreiro L, Nieto Serradilla L, et al. Efficacy of a continuous infusion of local anesthetic into the surgical wound for pain relief after abdominal hysterectomy. Rev Esp Anestesiol Reanim 2009;56(7):417–24 [in Spanish].

18. Forastiere E, Sofra M, Giannarelli D, et al. Effectiveness of continuous wound infusion of 0.5% ropivacaine by On-Q pain relief system for postoperative pain after open nephrectomy. Br J Anaesth 2008;101(6):841–7.

19. Sakellaris G, Petrakis I, Makatounaki K, et al. Effects of ropivacaine infiltration on cortisol and prolactin responses to postoperative pain after inguinal hernioraphy in children. J Pediatr Surg 2004;39(9):1400–3.
20. Matsota P, Papageorgio–Brousta M, Kostopanagiotou G. Wound Infiltration with levobupivacaine: an alternate method of postoperative pain relief after inguinal hernia repair in children. Eur J Pediatr Surg 2007;17(4):270–4.
21. Stelter K, Hempel JM, Berghaus A, et al. Application methods of local anesthetic infiltrations for postoperative pain relief in tonsillectomy: a prospective random-ized, double blind, clinical trial. Eur Arch Otorhinolaryngol 2009;266:1615–20.
22. Dagtekin O, Hotz A, Kampe S, et al. Postoperative analgesia and flap perfusion after pedicled TRAM flap reconstruction-continuous wound instillation with ropivacaine 0.2%. A pilot study. J Plast Reconstr Aesthet Surg 2009;62:618–25.
23. Legeby M, Jurell G, Beausang-Linder M, et al. Placebo-controlled trial of local anaesthesia for treatment of pain after breast reconstruction. Scand J Plast Reconstr Surg Hand Surg 2009;43:315–9.
24. Pacik PT, Nelson CE, Werner C. Pain control in augmentation mammoplasty: safety and efficacy of indwelling catheters in 644 consecutive patients. Aesthet Surg J 2008;28:279–84.
25. Johansson A, Kornfa J, Nordin L, et al. Wound infiltration with ropivacaine and fentanyl: effects on postoperative pain and PONV after breast surgery. J Clin Anesth 2003;15:113–8.
26. Rica MA, Norlia A, Rohaizak M, et al. Preemptive ropivacaine local anesthetic infiltration versus postoperative wound infiltration in mastectomy: postoperative pain and drain outputs. Asian J Surg 2007;30(1):34–9.
27. Marret E, Vigneau A, Salengro A, et al. Effectiveness of analgesic techniques after breast surgery: a meta analysis. Ann Fr Anesth Reanim 2006;25:947–54 [in French].
28. Bray DA Jr, Nguyen J, Craig J, et al. Efficacy of a local anesthetic pain pump in abdominoplasty. Plast Reconstr Surg 2007;119:1054–9.
29. Saringcarinkul A, Boonsri S. Effect of scalp infiltration on postoperative pain relief in elective supratentorial craniotomy with 0.5% bupivacaine with adrenaline 1:400,000. J Med Assoc Thai 2008;91(10):1518–23.
30. Gurbet A, Bekar A, Bilgin H, et al. Pre-emptive infiltration of levobupivacaine is superior to at-closure administration in lumbar laminectomy patients. Eur Spine J 2008;17:1237–41.
31. Gottschalk A, Burmeister MA, Radtke P, et al. Continuous wound infiltration with ropivacaine reduces pain and analgesic requirement after shoulder surgery. Anesth Analg 2003;97:1086–91.
32. Singelyn FJ, Lhotel L, Fabre B. Pain relief after arthroscopic shoulder surgery: a comparison of intraarticular analgesia, suprascapular nerve block, and inter-scalene brachial plexus block. Anesth Analg 2004;99:589–92.
33. Banerjee SS, Pulido P, Adelson WS, et al. The efficacy of continuous bupivacaine infiltration following arthroscopic rotator cuff repair. Arthroscopy 2008;24: 397–402.
34. Barber FA, Herbert MA. The effectiveness of an anesthetic continuous-infusion device on postoperative pain control. Arthroscopy 2002;18:76–81.
35. Boss AP, Maurer T, Seiler S, et al. Continuous subacromial bupivacaine infusion for postoperative analgesia after open acromioplasty and rotator cuff repair: preliminary results. J Shoulder Elbow Surg 2004;13:630–4.
36. Eroglu A. A comparison of patient-controlled subacromial and i.v. analgesia after open acromioplasty surgery. Br J Anaesth 2006;96:497–501.

37. Harvey GP, Chelly JE, AlSamsam T, et al. Patient controlled ropivacaine analgesia after arthroscopic subacromial decompression. Arthroscopy 2004;20:451–5.
38. Klein SM, Nielsen KC, Martin A, et al. Interscalene brachial plexus block with continuous intraarticular infusion of ropivacaine. Anesth Analg 2001;93:601–5.
39. Hansen BP, Beck CL, Beck EP, et al. Post arthroscopic glenohumeral chondrolysis. Am J Sports Med 2007;35:1628–34.
40. Bailie DS, Ellenbecker T. Severe chondrolysis after shoulder arthroscopy: a case series. J Shoulder Elbow Surg 2009;18:742–7.
41. Webb ST, Ghosh S. Intra-articular bupivacaine: potentially chondrotoxic? Br J Anaesth 2009;102:439–41.
42. Gomoll AH, Kang RW, William JM, et al. Chondrolysis after continuous intraarticular bupivacaine infusion: an experimental model investigating chondrotoxicity in the rabbit shoulder. The Journal of Arthroscopic and Related Surgery. Arthroscopy 2006;22(8):813–9.
43. Rapley JH, Beavis C, Barber FA. Glenohumeral chondrolysis after shoulder arthroscopy associated with continuous bupivacaine infusion. The Journal of Arthroscopic and Related Surgery. Arthroscopy 2009;25(12):1367–73.
44. Anderson L, Buchko JZ, Taillon MR, et al. Chondrolysis of the glenohumeral joint after infusion of bupivacaine through an intra-articular pain pump catheter: a report of 18 cases. The Journal of Arthroscopic and Related Surgery. Arthroscopy 2010;26(4):451–61.
45. Scheffel PT, Clinton J, Lynch JR, et al. Glenohumeral chondrolysis: a systematic review of 100 cases from the English language literature. J Shoulder Elbow Surg 2010;19:944–9.
46. Solomon DJ, Navaie M, Stedje-Larsen ET, et al. Glenohumeral chondrolysis after arthroscopy: a systematic review of potential contributors and causal pathways. The Journal of Arthroscopic and Related Surgery. Arthroscopy 2009;25(11):1329–42.
47. Busfield BT, Romero DM. Pain pump use after shoulder arthroscopy as a cause of glenohumeral chondrolysis. The Journal of Arthroscopic and Related Surgery. Arthroscopy 2009;25(6):647–52.
48. I-Flow Corporation. Available at: http://www.iflo.com/pdf/products/1305324a.pdf. Accessed August 12, 2009.
49. Kerr D, Kohan L. Local infiltration analgesia: a technique for the control of acute postoperative pain following knee and hip surgery. A case study of 325 patients. Acta Orthop 2008;79(2):174–83.
50. Mauerhan DR, Campbell M, Miller JS, et al. Intra-articular morphine and/or bupivacaine in the management of pain after total knee arthroplasty. J Arthroplasty 1997;12(5):546–52.
51. Dahl JB, Møiniche S, Kehlet H. Wound infiltration with local anaesthetics for postoperative pain relief. Acta Anaesthesiol Scand 1994;38:7–14.
52. Fredman B, Shapiro A, Zohar E, et al. The analgesic efficacy of patient controlled Ropivacaine installation after cesarean delivery. Anesth Analg 2000;91:1436–40.
53. Rømsing J, Møiniche S, Ostergaard D, et al. Local infiltration with NSAIDs for postoperative analgesia: evidence for a peripheral analgesic action. Acta Anaesthesiol Scand 2000;44:672–83.
54. Bianconi M, Ferraro L, Traina GC, et al. Pharmacokinetics and efficacy of ropivacaine continuous wound instillation after joint replacement surgery. Br J Anaesth 2003;91:830–5.
55. Röstlund T, Kehlet H. High-dose local infiltration analgesia after hip and knee replacement—what is it, why does it work, and what are the future challenges? Guest editorial. Acta Orthop 2007;78(2):159–61.

56. Andersen LJ, Poulsen T, Krogh B, et al. Postoperative analgesia in total hip arthro-plasty: a randomized double-blinded, placebo-controlled study on preoperative and postoperative ropivacaine, ketorolac, and adrenaline wound infiltration. Acta Orthop 2007;78(2):187–92.

57. Busch CA, Whitehouse MR, Shore BJ, et al. The efficacy of periarticular multimodal drug infiltration in total hip arthroplasty. Clin Orthop Relat Res 2010;468:2152–9.

58. Lombardi AV, Berend KR, Mallory TH, et al. Soft tissue and intra-articular injection of bupivacaine, epinephrine, and morphine has a beneficial effect after total knee arthroplasty. Clin Orthop Relat Res 2004;428:125–30.

59. Busch CA, Shore BJ, Bhandaril R, et al. Efficacy of periarticular multimodal drug injection in total knee arthroplasty a randomized trial. J Bone Joint Surg Am 2006; 88(5):959–63.

60. Toftdahl K, Nikolajsen L, Haraldsted V, et al. Comparison of peri- and intra-articular analgesia with femoral nerve block after total knee arthroplasty: a randomized clinical trial. Acta Orthop 2007;78:172–9.

61. Andersen LO, Husted H, Otte KS, et al. High volume infiltration analgesia in total knee arthroplasty: a randomized double-blind placebo-controlled trial. Acta Anaesthesiol Scand 2008;52:1331–5.

62. Essving P, Axelsson K, Kjellberg J, et al. Reduced hospital stay, morphine consumption, and pain intensity with local infiltration analgesia after unicompart-mental knee arthroplasty. Acta Orthop 2009;80(2):213–9.

63. Fu P, Wu Y, Wu H, et al. Efficacy of intra-articular cocktail analgesic injection in total knee arthroplasty. A randomized controlled trial. Knee 2009;16:280–4.

64. Essving P, Axelsson K, Kjellberg J, et al. Reduced morphine consumption and pain intensity with local infiltration analgesia (LIA) following total knee arthro-plasty. A randomized double-blind study involving 48 patients. Acta Orthop 2010;81(3):354–60.

65. Andersen LO, Husted H, Kristensen BB, et al. Analgesic efficacy of intracapsular and intra-articular local anaesthesia for knee arthroplasty. Anaesthesia 2010;64: 904–12.

66. Bengisun ZK, Salviz EA, Darcin K, et al. Intraarticular levobupivacaine or bupiva-caine administration decreases pain scores and provides a better recovery after total knee arthroplasty. J Anesth 2010;24:694–9.

67. Gomez-Cardero P, Rodrıguez-Merchan EC. Postoperative analgesia in TKA ropi-vacaine continuous intraarticular infusion. Clin Orthop Relat Res 2010;468: 1242–7.

68. Andersen LO, Husted H, Kristensen BB, et al. Analgesic efficacy of subcutaneous local anaesthetic wound infiltration in bilateral knee arthroplasty: a randomised, placebo-controlled, double-blind trial. Acta Anaesthesiol Scand 2010;54:543–8.

69. Carli F, Clemente A, Asenjo JF, et al. Analgesia and functional outcome after total knee arthroplasty: periarticular infiltration vs continuous femoral nerve block. Br J Anaesth 2010;105(2):185–95.

70. Andersen KV, Bak M, Christensen BV, et al. A randomized, controlled trial comparing local infiltration analgesia with epidural infusion for total knee arthro-plasty. Acta Orthop 2010;81(5):606–10.

71. Ziegler CM, Wiechnik J, Muhling J. Analgesic effects of intra-articular morphine in patients with temporomandibular joint disorders: a prospective, double-blind, placebo-controlled clinical trial. J Oral Maxillofac Surg 2010;68:622–7.

72. Likar R, Koppert W, Blatnig H, et al. Efficacy of peripheral morphine analgesia in inflamed, non-inflamed and perineural tissue of dental surgery patients. J Pain Symptom Manage 2001;21:330–7.

73. Fu PL, Xiao J, Zhu YL, et al. Efficacy of a multimodal analgesia protocol in total knee arthroplasty: a randomized, controlled trial. J Int Med Res 2010;38(4): 1404–12.

74. Mullaji A, Kanna R, Shetty GM, et al. Efficacy of periarticular injection of bupivacaine, fentanyl, and methylprednisolone in total knee arthroplasty a prospective, randomized trial. J Arthroplasty 2010;25(6):851–7.

75. Andersen LK, Kristensen BB, Madsen JL, et al. Wound spread of radiolabeled saline with multi/ versus few-hole catheters. Reg Anesth Pain Med 2010;35: 200–2.

Index

Note: Page numbers of article titles are in **boldface** type.

A

Abdominal surgery, wound infiltration analgesia for, 330–331
Acute pain, processing pathways of, 292–293
Acute pain management, challenges in, **291–309**
    acute pain processing pathways, 292–293
    elderly and cognitively impaired patients, 297–298
    hepatic disease, 302–303
    neuralgic disease, 301–302
    objective pain assessments in challenging patients, 293–303
    opioid tolerance in chronic pain patients, 294–296
    opioid-induced hyperalgesia, 293–294
    patient characteristics influencing management, 293–303
    renal disease, 302–303
    sickle cell disease, 297
    sleep apnea, 298–301
    substance abuse and addiction, 296–297
  new concepts in, **311–327**
  regional analgesia and, 179–342
    complications of, **257–278**
    economics and practice management issues with, **213–232**
    local anesthetic systemic toxicity, **233–242**
    local infiltration analgesia, **329–342**
    neuraxial, unintentional subdural injection with, **279–290**
    peripheral nerve blocks, continuous, in hospital or home, **193–211**
        outcomes of ultrasound-guided, **179–191**
    postblock neurologic injury, **243–256**
Addiction, as challenge for acute pain management, 296–297
Ambulatory infusion, for continuous peripheral nerve blocks in hospital and at
    home, 197–199
    discharge, 198
    home care, 198–199
    infusion pump selection, 197–198
Analgesia. *See* Local analgesia *and* Regional analgesia.
Analgesic gap, challenges in acute pain management, **291–309**
Anesthesiologists, education of, on ultrasound-guided regional anesthesia, 186–187
    impact on costs of acute pain management, 214–215
Anesthetized adults, regional anesthesia in, 273–274
Anticoagulated patients, hemorrhagic complications of plexus and peripheral
    blockade in, 266–267
Antihyperalgesics, to prevent chronic postsurgical pain, 321–323
Aseptic technique, to avoid infectious complications of regional anesthesia, 269–270

Anesthesiology Clin 29 (2011) 343–351
doi:10.1016/S1932-2275(11)00033-4
1932-2275/11/$ – see front matter © 2011 Elsevier Inc. All rights reserved.

anesthesiology.theclinics.com

Moving?

Make sure your subscription moves with you!

To notify us of your new address, find your **Clinics Account Number** (located on your mailing label above your name), and contact customer service at:

Email: journalscustomerservice-usa@elsevier.com

800-654-2452 (subscribers in the U.S. & Canada)
314-447-8871 (subscribers outside of the U.S. & Canada)

Fax number: 314-447-8029

Elsevier Health Sciences Division
Subscription Customer Service
3251 Riverport Lane
Maryland Heights, MO 63043